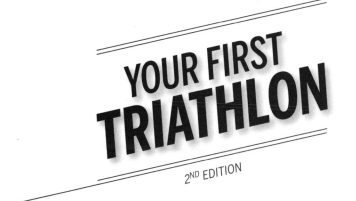

YOUR FIRST
TRIATHLON

2ND EDITION

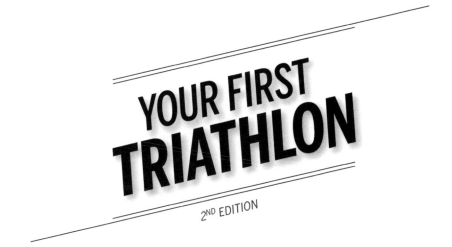

YOUR FIRST TRIATHLON

2ND EDITION

JOE FRIEL

BOULDER, COLORADO

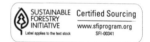

3002 Sterling Circle, Suite 100
Boulder, Colorado 80301-2338 USA
(303) 440-0601 · Fax (303) 444-6788 · E-mail velopress@competitorgroup.com

Distributed in the United States and Canada by Ingram Publisher Services

Library of Congress Cataloging-in-Publication Data
Friel, Joe.
Your first triathlon / Joe Friel.—2nd ed.
        p. cm.
Includes bibliographical references and index.
ISBN 978-1-934030-86-8 (pbk.)
I. Title.
GV1060.73.F75 2012
796.42'57—dc23

                        2012005121

For information on purchasing VeloPress books, please call (800) 811-4210 ext. 2138 or visit www.velopress.com.

This paper meets the requirements of
ANSI/NISO Z39.48-1992 (Permanence of Paper).

SUSTAINABLE FORESTRY INITIATIVE
Certified Sourcing
www.sfiprogram.org
SFI-00341
Label applies to the text stock

Cover design by Erin Johnson
Interior design and composition by Anita Koury
Cover and interior illustrations by Charlie Layton, except for pp. 92–94 by Todd Telander
Bike photographs courtesy of Specialized, pp. 67 and 71; Cannondale, p. 68; Trek, p. 69; and Pivot Cycles, p. 70.

Text set in Whitman 11/16.

12   13   14 / 10   9   8   7   6   5   4   3   2   1

To "Sunshine"—my granddaughter, Keara Friel,
who is training for her first triathlon

CONTENTS

5

6

7

8

9

ACKNOWLEDGMENTS

I want to thank the thousands of triathletes I have coached, consulted with, spoken to, and answered questions for over the past 31 years. They have provided the passion of triathlon. I also want to thank the many coaches with whom I have worked closely from the time, more than 20 years ago, when I found out about the *other* triathlon coach in the United States, to now, when there are thousands. They have provided the understanding of training for triathlon.

I especially want to thank Bob Hinkel, whom I met at LaCamas Swim and Sport in Camas, Washington, when I did a talk there for the members. For years Bob enlisted, encouraged, and assisted a group of budding triathletes preparing for their first races at various distances. The idea for this book came to me over dinner with Bob in February 2005.

INTRODUCTION

Welcome to the sport of triathlon!

You're about to embark on an exciting adventure that will improve your fitness, boost your health, and raise your self-esteem. Most of all, it will make your life richer and more enjoyable. While triathlon is fun, it is also challenging. In fact, it may well be the challenge that attracted you. Most new triathletes tell me that they came to the sport simply to see if they could do it—to challenge themselves. Once they tried it, they were hooked.

I'm sure that mastering three endurance sports and doing them all back-to-back, nonstop, seems like a rather daunting task. It should, but I'm sure you can do it. I've helped many people become triathletes over the past 25 years. With your motivation and my guidance, I'm certain you will do just fine. I have no doubt that, armed with the answers to basic questions and a dedication to training, you will successfully finish your first triathlon in a few weeks. That is the single purpose of this book— for you to cross the finish line with a smile on your face and become a triathlete.

Your First Triathlon provides the answers to many common triathlon questions:

How do I need to train?
What should I eat?
Do I need a new bike?
Which race should I enter?

Should I buy special triathlon clothing?

What happens at a triathlon?

Of course, there are hundreds of other questions you will have before your first race. Due to its inherent nature, blending three sports into one, triathlon is a complex undertaking. Most of your questions will be answered in the following pages, but there could be some left unresolved after you've read this book. Another resource you can use is my blog (joefrielsblog.com). Use the "search" function to look for key words in your question. If that doesn't help, feel free to send me an email (address listed on the blog page). One of my coaches will get back to you with an answer. Believe me, if you have a question, someone else has had that same question before, and I can help you with it.

Your First Triathlon gently guides you through the adventure of preparing for a sprint- or an Olympic-distance triathlon. In the first four chapters the basics of getting your lifestyle organized around triathlon training are discussed. This includes such topics as understanding the basics of the sport, setting goals, controlling body weight, eating for triathlon, and receiving outside support.

Chapters 5 through 8 cover the nuts and bolts of triathlon training—swimming, biking, and running. Here you'll also find simple ways to improve muscle strength and flexibility to avoid injuries and become more fit. Then we bring it all together in Chapter 9 with a training plan that fits your new lifestyle and your level of commitment. If you've just discovered this book and have your first triathlon coming up in 12 weeks or less, start with Chapter 9 so you can begin training right away. Then go back and read the supporting chapters.

Chapter 10 is a quick overview of some additional equipment you may want to consider buying to train more effectively. And finally, Chapter 11 gets you ready to go to your first triathlon feeling confident. Here you'll discover what to plan on for race day and before, how to dress, what exactly you need to bring with you, how to set up your transition area, and what to expect when swimming, biking, running, and finishing the race.

At the back of the book you will find other helpful information, including web and book resources, checklists, and a glossary of triathlon terms. Whenever you come across a term you don't understand, check out the Glossary in the back of the book. Appendix A will provide the details you need to do the workouts listed in Chapter 9.

All this information may seem a bit overwhelming. That's understandable; the sport of triathlon can be quite intimidating at first. But learning in small doses what to expect and what it takes to get there will make this challenge less daunting and more fun. And fun is what it's all about. Let's get started!

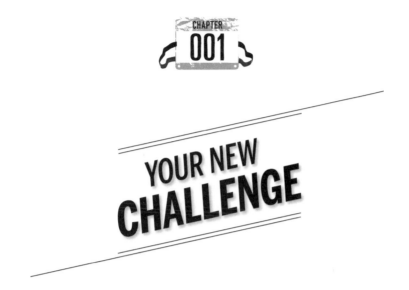

CHAPTER

001

YOUR NEW CHALLENGE

Why do you want to do a triathlon? Maybe it's because you've heard that exercise is good for you and that people who exercise regularly have a lower risk of heart disease, cancer, and other diseases, that they live longer and have a better quality of life. Or maybe it's because exercise has been shown to reduce stress, promote clear thinking and creativity, and build confidence.

Although these are all good reasons to take up triathlon, I'll bet you are thinking of doing a triathlon for far more pragmatic reasons. Chances are your friend registered for a race and has talked you into doing it also. Or it could be that triathlon is the new challenge that you've been looking for, a sport that will test your limits. There's no doubt that it will. Losing weight, looking better, and eating without guilt could be the things that are motivating you. Then again, maybe you just want to have fun. Triathlon can help you accomplish all this and more.

Regardless of your reason, you certainly want your first triathlon to go well, so you bought this book to find tips on how to prepare. You did the right thing. I've been coaching triathletes since the early days of the sport, and I've prepared many novices for their first races. I'm sure I can help you, too. This book is filled with advice that will guide you through the planning and training and ultimately across the finish line.

Let's start with the best advice I have to offer you: You should have only one goal for your first triathlon—to finish the race with a smile on your face. It doesn't matter what your time is or how you place in your age group or even if you are one of the last finishers. Just finish the race. Nothing else matters, other than the smile, of course. I've been saying this to new triathletes for more than 30 years. Those who follow my ad-

How Triathlon Got Its Start

In 1974 the San Diego Track Club added a short race to its calendar, a combination of running 4.8 miles, biking 5 miles, and swimming half a mile. All three sports were popular pastimes in Southern California, which was a natural fit for the birth of the sport.

In 1978 the first Ironman triathlon was held in Oahu, Hawaii, with 15 participants. The race was meant to determine who was the best athlete—the swimmer, the biker, or the runner. The athletes swam 2.4 miles at Waikiki Beach, biked 115 miles around the island, and ran a 26.2-mile marathon. The first winner, Gordon Haller, was a navy man and former pentathlete.

For the next 20 years the sport grew slowly but steadily, with a mix of both short- and long-distance races. In 1996 the international Olympic Committee announced that triathlon would be an Olympic sport in the 2000 Games in Sydney, Australia, a country that had also embraced triathlon. At the Sydney Olympics the women's triathlon was the first event, with the men's race the following day. I was there with Team USA and watched both races. The Australian crowd was incredibly enthusiastic about this "new" sport. Both events were televised around the world and created a lot of excitement for triathlon. Since then, triathlon has experienced phenomenal growth both in the United States and around the world.

vice have a lot of fun and a long triathlon career. Those who disregard it often don't finish their first triathlon, find themselves depressed afterward, and don't stay in the sport for very long. My purpose in this book is to help you accomplish this one simple goal. I will be coaching you, and I'm certain that, if you follow my advice, you will be successful.

RACE DISTANCES

Today there are four common triathlon distances. The longest, and the one most people think of when they hear the word "triathlon," is the Ironman-distance or "ultra-distance" race. Ironman is the most readily recognized race, probably because it gets the most press and has been around a long time. The swim is 2.4 miles (4,000 m) in open water, the bike portion is 112 miles (180 km), and the run is 26.2 miles (42.2 km). The winning times are generally about eight hours for the men and nine for the women. The last-finisher cutoff time is 17 hours.

The next-longest race distance is the half-Ironman or "long-course" race, with a 1.2-mile (2,000-m) open-water swim, a 56-mile (90-km) bike ride, and a 13.1-mile (21.1-km) run. It's sometimes called a "70.3" race since that's what the race distances in miles add up to. This is a very popular event among seasoned triathletes and is growing rapidly. The participants complete the race in about four to eight hours.

The Olympic-distance triathlon, sometimes called the "international-distance" race, dates back to the early 1980s and is the distance used today in Olympic and World Cup competitions. In these elite-only events the athletes are allowed to draft, or to follow closely behind each other, on the bike. In almost all the races done by amateurs, regardless of distance, drafting is not allowed. The Olympic-distance swim at 1,500 meters is just short of a mile, the bike leg is 25 miles (40 km), and the run is 6.2 miles (10 km). The pros generally complete the race in under two hours, with the last finishers taking up to five hours.

The shortest-distance triathlon is the "sprint" or "short-course" race. The typical sprint is a half-mile (750 m) swim, a 12.4-mile (20-km) bike ride, and a 3.1-mile (5-km) run, but the distances may be longer or shorter. The swim is often done in a pool, which makes it a good event for the triathlon newbie. Open water can be a bit intimidating to some novice swimmers. These races take one to two hours to complete, so they are hardly a real "sprint" except when compared with an Ironman.

You'll find that there are slight variations in these distances—especially the sprint—and that there are some races that don't fit neatly into any of these categories. There are also other combinations of the three sports, such as swim-run-bike and run-bike-swim. Run-bike-run races are called "duathlons" or sometimes "biathlons." Some cities have swim-run races, known officially by the tongue-twisting name "aquathlon" but usually called something like "splash and dash" or "stroke and stride." The distances for these sport variations are not standard, but they tend to be like the Olympic- or sprint-distance triathlons.

CHOOSING AND ENTERING A RACE

Selecting the right first race is as important as training for it. There's a real advantage to racing in your hometown because you might already know the course or at least have the opportunity to practice on it. Familiarity and easy logistics will give you a bit of a psychological boost and reduce the uneasiness you might otherwise feel on race day.

If you need help finding a race, go online to www.trifind.com. This search engine allows you to sort events by state and by race distance. You can also find a listing of triathlons for beginners, women, and kids. For an updated list of events sanctioned by USA Triathlon (USAT), check out their calendar at www.USATriathlon.org. Then select "short" (sprint distance) or "intermediate" (Olympic distance) along with preferred dates, location, and other details to view a list of all such races sanctioned by USAT.

You can sign up for many of these races online, and a link is provided to each on both the TriFind.com and USAT web sites. If the race you plan to participate in isn't listed, you may have to register locally or mail in your registration form.

Most races require a USA Triathlon racing license. Some small local events that aren't USA Triathlon–sanctioned don't require a license. You can purchase either a one-day license or one to cover the entire season. If you think you'll do more than one race this year, the seasonal license is the way to go. As of this writing a seasonal license costs $39— get yours at the USA Triathlon web site or at registration. Race-day-only licenses are always available when you register for the race. Expect to pay about $10. In either case, this will be made clear when you sign up for the race.

YOUR FIRST RACE

If you have decided on a race to enter, I hope it is a sprint- or Olympic-distance triathlon. The time commitment is less than five hours a week if you follow the training plan in Chapter 9. An Olympic triathlon will take a bit more time. Expect to work out about seven hours a week for this distance. With a day off each week to make sure you get enough rest, this works out to less than an hour a day for a sprint-distance race and about one hour each day for an Olympic-distance race. Of course, if you have more time than that, you can fit in more workouts. My training plans (found in the appendixes) include optional swim, bike, and run workouts each week to supplement your basic training.

If you hope to complete a longer triathlon on your first attempt, I advise you to reconsider. I've noticed that it's not uncommon for ambitious newcomers to choose an Ironman-distance race as their first triathlon. They jump at the chance to experience the ultimate challenge right away. Most athletes have no idea what they are up against and are in for a rude awakening. It may look easy on TV, but the difficulty of completing an Ironman on race day is well beyond what most could even imagine, and training for such an endeavor is like having a part-time job.

The best way to prepare for an Ironman-distance triathlon is to first do a sprint or an Olympic triathlon and then work your way up to completion of several Olympic races and a few half-Ironman events. Starting from the get-go with an Ironman can be devastating and typically leads to a very short tri career.

CAN YOU DO IT?

Attitude in sport is everything. If you believe in yourself and reinforce positive thinking habits daily, you will succeed. Your goal is to finish a triathlon—smiling. I know you can do it because I've seen many others succeed. In fact, I've never had anyone fail who followed the guidelines and training program I present here. I believe in you.

Others also believe you can do it. But there may be some who don't, and they may even tell you so. The most important opinion, however, is yours. Do you believe? What is the voice in your head saying about your chances of success as a triathlete? When it comes to success or failure in this sport, the voice in your head can be your strongest ally or your greatest enemy. You decide which it will be.

If you've trained the voice to find fault, you probably won't make it across that finish line. But if your self-talk is positive, success is practically ensured. Negative self-talk focuses your mind on the obstacles. And, rest assured, your mind will come up with plenty of obstacles to get you out of training: "I'm too busy to work out today." "I'm too tired to get up early." "I just don't feel like it." A positive attitude allows you to clearly see ways around such obstacles and keeps you on track.

Certainly there will be setbacks; that's the way life is. Instead of dwelling on what you could have done, look for the learning experience in every misfortune. The only difference between winning and losing in triathlon, as in life, is that when we fail, we learn something—or at least we should.

Imagine how boring and unfulfilling life would be without obstacles. Where would the thrill of victory come from were it not for the agony of defeat? Obstacles are good. Accept them while focusing on their challenges, and you will enjoy satisfaction and fulfillment in triathlon and in life. Wallow in them, and you will ensure defeat. Some opposition is always necessary for attainment. Kites rise against, not with, the wind.

Defeat in whatever form is often blamed on physical obstacles, such as lack of some physical ability, like endurance, strength, or speed. The negative thinker sees this obstacle as insurmountable. The positive athlete instead sees two opportunities: taking advantage of known strengths and learning about weaknesses so that they can be improved upon. Endurance, strength, and speed can all be developed.

What if you don't see the opportunities? Start by recognizing your shortcomings and being open to change. This is 90 percent of what it takes to cultivate a positive attitude. The final 10 percent comes with positive reinforcement, practiced daily. Here's a strategy to get you on the right track: Every night when you go to bed, between the time when the lights go out and you fall asleep, review your greatest success of the day, no matter how trivial. Perhaps you completed a workout that was difficult; relive that accomplishment. It could even be something as seemingly minor as starting a workout when motivation was low. Remember the success. Mentally celebrate the victory. Look for and relive your successes every day, and your attitude and belief in yourself will improve. I've advised every athlete I've coached, from newbie to Olympian, to adopt this strategy. It works.

A NEW SPORT (OR THREE)

In the early days of the sport (ca. 1983), most of those doing a first triathlon were injured runners. That's how I got started. Every time I'd break down while training for the next marathon, I'd get my bike out of the garage and ride it. Then one day I had a bad bike accident and broke my shoulder. The doctor said one of the best ways to rehabilitate it was swimming. While I was in the pool one day after the shoulder had healed, it dawned on me that I was swimming, biking, and running, so why not try out that new sport—triathlon? I did and was hooked.

Things have changed since then. Most people who are new to triathlon don't have a background in another sport. For them triathlon is their first and only sport. Part of the attraction of triathlon for newcomers is that it's a bit like being a kid again, with lots of variety and options. It's fun to alternate among swimming, biking, and running instead of being stuck with one sport. What better way to seek a brief escape from the daily chores and responsibilities of life than to head to the pool or to go out on the road?

Your friends and family might not share this sentiment. Most outside observers see triathletes as masochists and can't imagine why anyone would want to do such a thing. That's probably due to the sport's roots and Julie Moss's famous crawl to the finish line in the Hawaii Ironman® in 1982. The media still foster this image of the "gruelathon," of participants "pushing the limits of human endurance" and fighting through unbelievable suffering as they struggle to the finish. It really isn't like that.

Don't get me wrong—triathlon is hard work. You won't get fit in three sports without dedication and perseverance. Although you've probably done harder things, this will rank right up there with some of the bigger challenges of your life. It will also be one of the most fun challenges you've ever taken on.

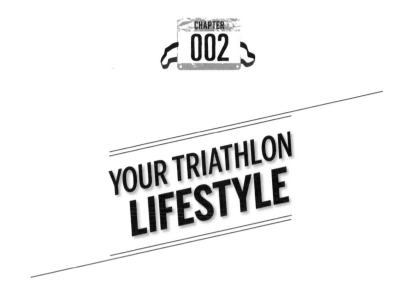

CHAPTER

002

YOUR TRIATHLON LIFESTYLE

Preparing for your first triathlon will demand a lot of you. First and foremost, it requires dedication. How are you going to fit swimming, biking, and running into your already busy life? The goal of finishing a triathlon is a worthy one, but the reality is that your free time is quite limited. It won't be easy at first; you might miss some workouts due to other commitments. On those days you will question whether you can be fit and ready by race day.

Despite the inevitable setbacks, there is no doubt that you can do it if you fully commit to your goal. You must also accept that you are not perfect and that there will be days when things don't go right. Even experienced triathletes miss workouts due to other important responsibilities; however, missing a workout must be a rare occurrence rather than a common one if you are to become a triathlete.

Consistency is key to success. Exercise needs to become the focal point of each and every day. Everything you do and when you do it must be determined by your next workout. This includes eating, working, preparing meals, mowing the lawn, and tackling hobbies and all other interests. The successful triathlete decides when the next workout will be and then arranges the other details of life around it.

This may sound obsessive—and I suppose it is to some extent—but what appears as obsession to one person is passion to another. If you want to finish your first triathlon in a few weeks, you need to be dedicated to exercising and maintaining a healthy lifestyle. This level of commitment is a whole lot easier if you are having fun. If you don't enjoy swimming, biking, and running, chances are that you will never make it to the start line, let alone to the finish line. Remember that your goal is to finish smiling.

Several other factors affect your triathlon success, including your level of motivation, recovery, health, weight, and age. Fortunately most of these are things that fall under your control, and with a little extra effort you can work each one to your advantage as a triathlete.

MOTIVATION

There will be times when you ask yourself, "Why am I doing this?" It's easy to say you're going to train for a triathlon; it's another thing entirely to drive to the pool at 5:30 a.m. or to hop on your bike before the sun rises. While most people are sleeping in on Saturday morning, you'll be working out. Unlike your coworkers who go home after work to drink a beer and watch TV, you'll head home to get your run in before dinner.

Success in triathlon depends heavily on motivation. It isn't going to be easy, but that's part of embracing the challenge. Preparing for your first triathlon means incorporating a self-improvement program into your already busy life. More than half the people who start an exercise program quit within a few weeks. What can you do to stay motivated during the weeks leading up to your first triathlon?

Stay the Course

Start by following the training plan laid out in Chapter 9. This eliminates one stumbling block—what to do each day. Just follow the plan. Know that there will be days when you miss a workout; that happens to all triathletes. It's nothing new. Just stick with the plan and focus on your next workout. Missed workouts should be the exception rather than the rule, but don't be too hard on yourself if this happens.

On the other hand, if you find yourself looking for reasons not to work out, it may be time for a gut check. To maintain motivation, continually remind yourself why you want to do a triathlon. Recall the benefits of training every day: You are keeping your weight and blood pressure down, strengthening your heart and muscles, improving your flexibility, building greater stamina, looking fit and trim, and feeling good about yourself. Envision what it will be like when you cross that finish line on race day, having achieved a major goal in your life. There is nothing quite like this feeling of euphoria and accomplishment. Do this mental drill whenever you see your resolve flagging.

For some it helps to visualize the effects of not continuing to work out regularly: further loss of fitness, possible weight gain, increasingly weak

Tips for Fitting in Workouts

Here are some other strategies that may help you stay on track:

- Exercise first thing in the morning, when there are fewer demands on your time. This is what most serious triathletes do.
- Schedule workouts in a weekly calendar as you would other appointments—and treat them like important appointments.
- Exercise with a friend; support (or peer pressure) encourages participation.
- Lay out exercise clothes and equipment the night before your workout. Knowing what you're going to wear makes it easy to get started in the morning.
- Ride a wind trainer or stationary bike while watching TV or reading. This makes great use of your valuable time.

and inflexible muscles, more rapid aging, and a greater risk for heart disease and cancer. Fear can be a good motivator, though in the long run a positive attitude and realistic goals will take you far.

Give Yourself Five Minutes

Here's a helpful strategy that I know many athletes, even the pros, find useful. If you just don't feel like exercising, tell yourself you will only do it for five minutes and then stop. This will get you out the door, and once into it you'll probably finish the workout. But if you still don't feel up to it after five minutes, call it quits and head home. It just isn't your day. Your body is probably trying to tell you something. Be sure to rest well and strengthen your resolve for tomorrow.

Remember that you are forming new habits, and that takes time. Don't be discouraged if you find that the triathlon lifestyle doesn't come easily and that on some days exercise is the last thing you want to do. At these times you must consciously decide that your goal is important and re-commit to achieving it. Overcoming the temptation to avoid exercise will make you a stronger person and, ultimately, a triathlete.

RECOVERY

Sometimes even new triathletes go too far with their passion for the sport. When pressed for time and feeling the need to fit in a workout or other activity, the first thing most triathletes do is cut back on sleep. They get up earlier or go to bed later in order to wedge more into each day. The problem with "creating" time in this way is that it compromises recovery and adaptation. During rest, especially sleep, the body mends and grows stronger. While you're sleeping, a growth hormone is released, producing a more physically fit body. If the time spent snoozing is shortened, it takes longer to recover. This compromises consistency, which is the single most important aspect of training.

Reducing sleep time also means that energy stores aren't fully replenished between workouts, leading to a drop in endurance performance over several days. The body's cells that are routinely damaged by strenuous exercise will take longer to repair, increasing the risk of injury and illness. If the training workload remains high despite decreased sleep time, overtraining becomes a real threat. Mental burnout is also waiting just around the corner for the triathlete who cuts back on sleep.

If you feel the need to make more time available for training, instead of cutting back on sleep, look for time wasters in your day and replace them. Perhaps the greatest time waster in most of our lives is television. Serious triathletes have one thing in common—they don't watch much TV.

A well-rested triathlete looks forward to the next workout, enjoys training, is powerful, has good endurance, and progressively grows stronger. A tired triathlete realizes none of these benefits. Never underestimate your need for sleep. The average person typically needs seven or eight hours of sleep every day. As a triathlete, you may need more. As you gradually increase the amount of exercise you're doing, stress will increase, as

Sleep Your Way to Better Fitness

Here are seven tips to improve the quality of your sleep:

1. Go to bed at a regular time every night.

2. Take a warm bath before bed.

3. Darken the room in the last hour before bedtime and narrow your focus by reading or engaging in light conversation.

4. Sleep in a dark, well-ventilated room that is 60–64 degrees Fahrenheit.

5. Systematically contract and relax each muscle group to induce total body relaxation.

6. Avoid stimulants such as coffee and tea in the last several hours before going to bed.

7. Restrict alcohol intake (which interferes with sleep patterns) at least a few hours prior to retiring.

will the need for slumber. And hours of sleep are not the only issue here; quality of sleep is just as important.

Triathlon training is much more than simply sweating and breathing hard while swimming, biking, and running. Training also depends heavily on adequate rest. By placing as much importance on sleep as on exercise, you will improve your training consistency as the quality of your workouts rises. The result is better fitness and success as a triathlete.

WEIGHT AND EXERCISE

According to the U.S. Centers for Disease Control and Prevention, today the average American man weighs 191 pounds and the average American woman tips the scales at 164 pounds. Each is carrying in the neighborhood of 25–30 pounds of excess body fat. There is little doubt that this unneeded weight has dire consequences for health. Diabetes, heart disease, and other deadly lifestyle diseases have been linked to obesity, which is officially defined as being 30 pounds or more over one's ideal body weight.

Of less importance but certainly related is the impact of excess body weight on triathlon performance. It's been estimated that each pound of additional body fat causes a runner to slow by two seconds per mile and requires an additional 1½ watts of power when climbing a hill on a bike. For the novice triathlete who is 25 pounds overweight, this means, in theory, taking 7–8 percent longer to finish a race, or about an extra 8–10 minutes in a sprint-distance event—double that for an Olympic-distance race. In actuality, it could be more than just a few minutes; a person this overweight will probably end up walking most of the run portion because his or her aerobic fitness will be inadequate to move that much mass at a running pace.

Do you need to shed a few pounds? If so, you've already taken a giant step in that direction by deciding to do a triathlon. Considerable research shows that regular exercise helps to control and reduce body fat. Exercise burns between 5 and 20 calories per minute depending on the type of exercise and its intensity. By exercising several times a week you will be burning additional calories and working your way toward a slimmer body, better triathlon performances, and improved long-term health. Controlling your eating can accelerate the process of losing excess luggage.

Do I Need a Physical?

The American College of Sports Medicine (ACSM) offers the following questions to help you decide if you should schedule a complete physical before starting a triathlon training program. If you answer yes to one or more of these questions, ACSM recommends that you consult with your doctor before starting an exercise program or increasing your current level of exercise.

1. Has your doctor ever told you that you have a heart condition?
2. Do you feel pain in your chest when you do physical activity?
3. Have you ever had a heart murmur that a physician considered significant?
4. In the past month, have you had chest pain when you were not doing physical activity?
5. Have you ever had pain, pressure, or a squeezing feeling in your chest that came on during exercise or other physical activity?
6. Do you lose balance because of dizziness or do you ever lose consciousness?
7. If you climb a few flights of stairs fairly rapidly, do you have tightness or a pressing pain in your chest?
8. Have you experienced problems breathing while exercising?
9. Do you have a bone or joint problem that could be made worse by a change in your physical activity?
10. Is your doctor currently prescribing drugs (e.g., water pills) for your blood pressure or a heart condition?
11. Do you know any other reason why you should not participate in a physical activity?
12. Has it been longer than 12 months since your last physical?

I know you've heard all this before, and if you're like most people, you've been on weight-loss diets and even tried exercising. You probably shed some pounds, but they came back with gusto. So why should it work this time?

For one thing, by following through on your goal to become a triathlete, you'll be changing your lifestyle. This won't be just another diet; it will be a new way of seeing exercise, food—and yourself. The difference is attitude and commitment. Triathletes as a whole are lean and fit. By adopting the triathlon lifestyle, you can be, too.

Successful Losers

When trying to understand weight loss the place to start is with those who have successfully lost weight and kept it off. In 1993, researchers at Brown University and Miriam Hospital in Providence, Rhode Island, established the National Weight Control Registry to keep track of people who lose at least 30 pounds and keep it off for at least one year. The people listed in the registry lost an average of 70 pounds and kept it off for six years. Several thousand people are listed in the registry and are studied by the researchers.

A great deal has been learned about successful weight loss from this research. For example, nearly 90 percent of those in the registry used a combination of exercise and reduced caloric intake to lose weight. Most of the women in the study relied heavily on walking for exercise. Men were more likely to run and lift weights. Participants burned, on average, 2,840 calories per week, or about 400 per day, through exercise, with the men's rate a bit higher than the women's. This amounts to about 4 miles of walking or running each day.

Participants reported eating an average of 1,387 calories daily, with men reporting more than women. This number may be low, as other studies have shown that people tend to underestimate their food intake by as much as 20 percent. If that is true here, then these folks may have been taking in closer to 1,664 calories daily.

You may be wondering how they could lose weight if they were burning 400 calories a day through exercise but taking in 1,664. The answer is found in their resting metabolic rate (RMR).

Calories Out

Resting metabolic rate is the amount of energy the body uses to maintain itself while lying down or sitting. RMR is increased by having greater muscle mass, increasing ambient air temperature, being young, having a higher body temperature, experiencing stress, and having certain hormones present. But here's the great part: Exercise causes RMR to rise after a workout. This post-exercise "burn" can account for a few hundred additional calories used daily.

RMR usually makes up about 60–75 percent of a person's total daily energy expenditure, with the remainder coming from exercise and normal movement at work, school, and home. Interestingly, eating also raises the RMR by as much as 10 percent because digesting food burns calories. The type of food that causes the greatest increase in RMR is protein. Protein is also the most satiating nutrient, and it's wise to include it in every meal and even with snacks.

You can get a rough estimate of your RMR by multiplying your body weight in pounds by 10. A 160-pound person would have an RMR of roughly 1,600 calories per day. To know that person's total daily energy expenditure, we would need to know how much normal activity he or she does in a day, plus calories burned during exercise, and add this to RMR. See Tables 2.1 and 2.2 to estimate your energy expenditure.

To estimate your total daily energy expenditure, use the following equation:

Total daily energy expenditure = A + B + C

A = RMR calories

B = Calories burned during normal daily activity

C = Calories burned during exercise

Table 2.1 Calories Burned During Daily Activities*

INTENSITY	EXAMPLES	CALORIES/MINUTE
Light	Working on computer, sitting at desk, watching TV	Included in RMR
Moderate	Gardening, standing, housecleaning, shopping	3–6
Heavy	Digging, shoveling snow, climbing stairs	7–9
Extreme	Lifting and carrying heavy loads	10–12

*Use this table to estimate how many calories you burn per minute beyond RMR throughout your daily activities, not including exercise or rest.

Table 2.2 Calories Burned During Exercise*

SPORT	CALORIES/MINUTE	CALORIES/DISTANCE
Swimming	10	5/25 yards
Biking	10	45/1 mile
Walking briskly	6	90/1 mile
Running	11	110/1 mile
Lifting weights vigorously	8	—

*This table allows you to roughly estimate the calories you burn during exercise. Actual numbers will vary with body size and intensity. These numbers include the RMR calories that are used during exercise.

Calories In

Now that you have an idea of how many calories you burn in a day, one of the keys to weight loss is to eat fewer than that daily. This is typically referred to as "calorie counting" and is a critical part of the National Weight Control Registry participants' strategy. Purchase a food and calorie book at your local drugstore or, better yet, use computer software to more easily manage your counting. You can find one designed for athletes at www.trainingpeaks.com.

In order to lose weight, registry members created a caloric deficit each day of about 500–800 calories. In other words, their average total daily energy expenditure including RMR and all daily activities was about 2,200–2,500 calories, while they ate just 1,700 calories. Theoretically, a

500-calorie daily deficit would result in the loss of one pound a week of body fat. An 800-calorie deficit would do it in just under five days.

I have often found such a rapid rate of weight loss to be counterproductive for athletes because recovery after workouts is compromised, leading to lower-quality exercise and even forced days off due to excessive fatigue. Reducing your food intake makes you tired in much the same way that exercise does. Missed workouts due to being tired mean a loss of fitness. I have had more success with athletes keeping their deficits at 300–500 calories daily. At this rate a pound of fat should come off every 7–12 days, with fewer negative consequences for recovery from daily exercise. Using the lower rate of loss, which is easier to maintain and less of an emotional burden, you would drop 7 pounds during the 12-week plans in Chapter 9. This amounts to 28 pounds in a year and could do wonders for your health and for triathlon performances in the future.

While it takes real dedication to lose weight, I suggest *not* reducing calories by this amount week after week for months on end. Your body—and your mind—needs occasional breaks from such a strictly disciplined lifestyle. Just as with Chapter 9's exercise plan, there need to be frequent "rest" weeks. After two or three weeks of reduced daily calories, give yourself a break for a week by allowing a few more calories. But do not go beyond your total daily energy exposure. After the rest week, return to restricting your calories. Once you've attained a reasonable body-weight goal, go back to normal—and healthy—eating. In the long term, by taking occasional breaks you will lose more weight and you'll also be happier. Both are important to your new triathlon lifestyle.

Should I Eat Less or Exercise More?

What is the best way for an athlete to lose weight? Unfortunately, few studies of serious athletes have looked at this question.

One group of researchers, however, has examined the issue in an interesting way. They compared eating less with exercising more to see which was more effective in eliminating excess body fat. They had six endurance-trained men create a 1,000-calorie-per-day deficit for seven days by either exercising more while maintaining their caloric intake or eating less while keeping their exercise the same. With 1,000 calories of increased exercise daily—comparable to running an additional 9 miles or so each day—the men averaged 1.67 pounds of weight loss in a week. The subjects eating 1,000 fewer calories each day lost 4.75 pounds on average for the week. So, according to this study, the old adage that "a calorie is a calorie" doesn't hold true. At least in the short term, restricting food intake appears to have a greater return *on the scales* than does increasing training workload. However, the reduced-food-intake group in this study unfortunately lost a greater percentage of muscle mass than did the increased-exercise group. That is an *ineffective* way to lose weight. If the scales show you're lighter, but you have less muscle to create power, then the trade-off is not a good one.

How can you reduce the calories you eat and yet maintain muscle mass? Unfortunately that question hasn't been answered for athletes, but it has been for sedentary women. Perhaps the conclusions are also applicable to athletes.

In 1994, Italian researchers had 25 women eat only 800 calories a day for 21 days. Ten ate a relatively high-protein and low-carbohydrate diet. Fifteen ate a low-protein and high-carbohydrate diet. Both were restricted to 20 percent of calories from fat. The two groups lost similar amounts of weight, but there was a significantly greater loss of muscle on the high-carbohydrate, low-protein diet.

It appears that when calories are reduced to lose weight, the protein content of the diet must be kept at near-normal levels. This assumes, of course, that you're eating adequate protein before starting the diet, which many athletes aren't. When you're training hard, a quality source of protein should be included in every meal, especially when you're trying to lose weight.

What If It Isn't Working?

Realize that the extra weight might not melt away as quickly as you'd like it to. There will even be those frustrating days—even weeks—when you stay at the same weight or regain weight despite continuing to watch what and how much you eat. These "plateaus" can be very frustrating and can tempt you to throw in the towel. Don't do it! Hang in there. The body is fickle about how it gives up its precious fat stores. Its first response to reduced calories is to slow down the resting metabolic rate. Regular meals and daily exercise will cause it to recalibrate. Be patient; this is a long-term project, so don't expect to weigh less every day.

Also, keep in mind that plenty of good is still happening on the inside when you are going through a dietary change combined with regular exercise. For one thing, while you are losing fat you are probably also gaining muscle. Since muscle weighs more than fat, the scales don't accurately reflect what is happening inside you.

Here are some other benefits of combining exercise with healthy eating:

Improved cardiovascular health. Exercise combined with healthy eating decreases your risk of heart disease (the number 1 killer in the United States) by lowering blood pressure and bad cholesterol.

Lower stress levels. Exercise and nutritious foods help you put the stresses of life into perspective and make for a calmer demeanor, which has been linked with better health.

Stronger immune system. When you exercise regularly and moderately while eating more healthfully, your body is better able to ward off disease.

Increased energy. A fit body stores more energy, meaning that you have more options in your daily life.

Stronger bones. Exercise and a sound diet help you prevent osteoporosis and the risk of broken bones, both of which typically come with aging.

When you next step on the scales or measure your waist, realize that these numbers aren't telling you the whole story. There are lots of good things happening inside that aren't always reflected in the mirror.

Daily Eating Strategies

The following are some strategies you can use to keep your calories in lower than your calories out:

Buy groceries with a plan in mind. When putting together your shopping list, decide what foods you will eat in the coming week. Do not buy foods that are not on the list. (Chapter 3 will help you with these shopping decisions.)

Keep a record of your daily calories in and out. Computer software and applications are very helpful for this, but a calorie-counting book and a notebook will work just as well.

Eat a lot of high-fiber, low-calorie foods. Good examples are fibrous fruits and vegetables. These will contribute to a feeling of satisfaction. Avoid low-fiber, high-calorie foods such as refined starches and sugars.

Reduce the variety of foods at a meal. Research reveals that having lots of choices at a meal causes people to eat more by as much as 25 percent. A meal should be no more than three food types. An example of such a meal is a lean protein (fish, shellfish, poultry), a vegetable (other than white) or a garden salad, and fruit or berries for dessert.

Stop when you're satisfied, not stuffed. Pay attention to how you feel while eating and stop when you are no longer hungry. Don't "clean your plate" as you were taught to do as a child. Slow down and pay attention to your body while eating. Set the fork down while you chew. Take your time; this is not the time to race.

Choose smaller portions. You can always add more if necessary, but having excess on your plate encourages continued eating even if you're no longer hungry. This is more difficult to do when eating out, since serving portions are decided for you. Remind yourself when you go to a restaurant that you don't have to eat everything on your plate.

Include your favorite unhealthy foods—occasionally. Registry participants actually binged at times. About one day a month they consumed a lot of calories. A few even did this weekly by having a food they wouldn't otherwise eat. Occasionally eating a pizza or a bowl of ice cream does not mean you have failed. "Occasionally" is the key word here.

Monitor weight daily. Registry participants weighed themselves daily to stay in touch with how they were doing. It serves not only as a gauge of progress but also as a daily reminder.

Don't skip meals. Only 4 percent of those in the registry indicated that they skipped meals. Nearly all ate three meals a day.

EXERCISE AND AGING

In my work as a coach I spend my days talking with some very fit people. So just like the doctor who knows how to spot the symptoms of sickness, when I meet strangers, I often speculate about how fit they are. Too often it's easy to see at a glance. Why are so many of us in bad shape? The reasons are obvious: poor food choices, overeating, smoking, excessive alcohol consumption, and lack of exercise.

We were born to be athletic and healthy. Most of the degeneration we associate with aging actually results from lack of use. We let our bodies rust out instead of wearing them out. Weak muscles, weight gain, reduced capacity for physical work, and even life-threatening health issues such as heart disease, some cancers, and high blood pressure can be avoided simply by being physically active and eating well. The problem is that we expect these changes to occur as we get older. When they occur, we see them as inevitable. They aren't.

Low fitness, poor health, obesity, and disease are not normal. Studies of our Stone Age ancestors, who lived more than 10,000 years ago, before the advent of civilization, reveal that they didn't suffer from such maladies even though they did not have a food pyramid, health clubs, personal trainers, or coaches. They ate what was readily available and used their bodies vigorously to cope with the demands of daily life. Even just a few decades ago our health concerns were far different than they are today.

This isn't to say you'll live forever by exercising regularly. A comedian once quipped that his otherwise healthy and ever-exercising grandfather was in the hospital "dying of nothing." But that's not the point. The issue here isn't quantity of life, but rather quality. Life is more enjoyable when you have the capacity to enjoy a wide variety of activities and are free of disease even into what we consider to be old age.

Age also isn't the issue. A study of 80- and 90-year-olds showed that strength and fitness gains can be made at any age given an appropriate program. Hundreds of senior citizens complete marathons, triathlons, and other athletic feats that many younger people consider impossible for themselves. It's all too common for people over 50 or 60 years of age to think they are "too old" to exercise regularly. That's preposterous. What is holding people back is motivation, not age. You can't turn back time to reverse your chronological age, but biological age is fully within your control. The secret to slowing the aging process is regular exercise.

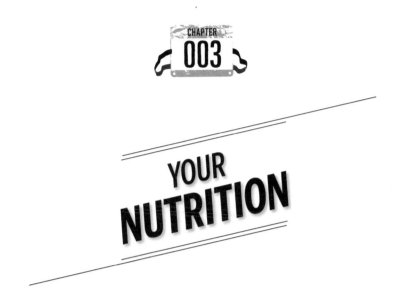

YOUR NUTRITION

Many factors determine how well prepared you are for your first triathlon. The three most important are your workouts, sleep, and nutrition. In Chapter 2, we discussed the necessity of adequate sleep in order for your body to properly recover. Chapters 5–9 and Appendixes B–F focus on your workouts and training plan—what to do for exercise and when to do it. That leaves nutrition.

What you eat and when you eat it play big roles in fitness. Food is fuel for your body. The experienced triathlete knows that high-quality foods, when eaten in the proper amounts at the right times, make workouts better, speed recovery after a hard workout, and ultimately contribute to better fitness. This doesn't mean these athletes never splurge and have a slice of pizza, a sugary soft drink, or even a doughnut. Each of us has a weakness for certain less-than-healthy foods. For me it's warm brownies, especially fresh from the oven. It's not a matter of *if* I will eat them, but *when*.

When to eat certain types of food is very important for triathlete nutrition. From a triathlon perspective, exercise is the most important aspect of your day. Decisions about what to eat must be made based on this daily event more than any other. With this in mind, there are four times, or "phases," in your day related to what you eat: right before exercise, during exercise, immediately after exercise, and throughout the rest of the day. In this chapter we examine the best foods to eat during each of the four phases. (For greater detail on this subject, see my book with Loren Cordain, *The Paleo Diet for Athletes*, 2nd ed. [Rodale Books, 2012].)

FUELING BEFORE EXERCISE

Exercising first thing in the morning may be the best time of day for you, as this is when there are few interruptions. Furthermore, scientific studies have shown that people who exercise in the morning are more regular and consistent than those who exercise at any other time of the day. So morning workouts are great for getting in shape.

But morning workouts can be problematic. For one thing, you may be groggy when you first awake and find it hard to get going. You may have to force yourself to move along more quickly in the morning, going faster than your legs or arms are prepared to go. In addition, some coaches and athletes believe that your risk of running injuries may be higher in the morning. The warm-up takes longer, so the stress on your joints, muscles, and tendons could be greater.

Another problem with morning workouts is eating. In a perfect world you'd have something to eat about two hours before starting to exercise. This not only would provide fuel for the workout but also would allow enough time for digestion. During the night, some of your body's carbohydrate stores were used up providing fuel for breathing, pumping your heart, moving around in the bed, and supporting other physiological demands of staying alive. If that fuel isn't at least partially replaced, you may feel even more sluggish and low on energy. But you certainly aren't going to get out of bed two hours early just because of this.

It may seem like a good idea to get up, eat some form of carbohydrates such as cereal, a bagel, or toast, read the paper for a few minutes while sipping a cup of coffee, and then head out the door to swim, bike, or run.

But with less than an hour or so before your workout, digestion won't be given a chance to do its thing. You may feel bloated, uncomfortable, and even a bit light-headed a few minutes into your workout.

The light-headed feeling results from how the body reacts to starchy foods. It pumps insulin into the bloodstream to move the sugar from the foods you just ate into your muscles and liver to restock the stores depleted during the night. But when insulin is faced with a flood of sugar from starchy foods, it tends to overreact and aggressively removes nearly all sugar from the blood, leaving you hypoglycemic—low on blood sugar. And since your brain uses sugar as its primary fuel source, when there isn't much available, you feel light-headed.

One way to resolve this problem is to take in nothing but water or unsweetened coffee or tea until 10 minutes before you start exercising. As you're putting on your swim goggles, pumping up your tires, or lacing up your running shoes, sip a sports drink or take some gel with water. But be sure to start your workout no more than 10 minutes after you consume the sports drink or gel. Ten minutes is not enough time for the body to send insulin out to do its job, so you start the workout with a few more calories in your body and no drop in blood sugar. Once exercise begins, the body deals with sugar in a different way, so insulin no longer presents a problem.

If you are not one to exercise first thing in the morning, you can eat something a couple of hours before the workout with little possibility of a downside. This could be a light meal with an emphasis on carbohydrates, especially from fruits and vegetables. If your stomach tends to be a bit squeamish during exercise even with a couple of hours separating your meal and your swim, bike, or run, you may need to eat pre-workout foods that are soft, low in fiber, and easily digested, such as unsweetened applesauce, bananas, sports-food supplements (e.g., GatorPro), liquid meals in a bottle (e.g., Ensure), and sports bars or blocks with water. I've even known triathletes to eat baby food, which is easy to digest. Many options exist when it comes to the combination of food and exercise, and finding foods that work for you is key to pre-workout eating.

Once you discover the right foods, stick with them. Warning signs that you haven't found the right foods or that you're eating too close to your workouts are an upset stomach, diarrhea, light-headedness, low energy, or early fatigue during exercise. Be aware that simply eating too much may also cause these symptoms, even if you ate two hours prior to exercise. About 400 calories, give or take a few depending on your size and tolerance for food first thing in the morning, is about right. If you eat less than two hours before exercise, reduce the calories. A rule of thumb is to eat about 200 calories for each hour before you begin working out. See Table 3.1 for sample pre-workout foods that may work for you before workouts and races, along with their caloric content.

Table 3.1 Fueling Before a Workout

		CALORIES
WHOLE FOODS	Applesauce, unsweetened (1 cup)	194
	Banana (1 medium)	105
	Oatmeal (1 packet)	104
	Potato, baked (1 medium)	220
	Fruit smoothie (12 oz.)	200–400
SPORTS DRINKS	EAS Myoplex Plus (16 oz.)	280
	Endura Optimizer (12 oz.)	280
	Endurox R4 (12 oz.)	280
	Ensure (8 oz.)	250
	GatorPro (11 oz.)	370
	Metabolol II (12 oz.)	260
	Met-Rx Original (16 oz.)	60
	OptiFuel 2 (12 oz.)	480
SPORTS BARS	Balance Bar	190
	Clif Builder's Bar	270
	Met-Rx Protein Plus	330
	PowerBar Pria	110

Chapter 11 addresses eating on the morning of your race. But in general, your stomach is likely to be a bit unsettled before an event, so the aforementioned easily digested foods are good options. Experimenting with them before workouts helps you identify what will work best at race time.

FUELING DURING EXERCISE

During exercise the body has two primary sources of fuel—its onboard stores of fat and carbohydrates. Each of us has plenty of fat and would gladly use it for fuel. But the body likes to save its fat, only increasing its reliance on that "tank" as the duration of your exercise increases. The less fit you are, the more it avoids burning fat. As you get in better aerobic shape, more fat is used for fuel during exercise. As the old saying goes, "The rich get richer and the poor get poorer!"

So when you first start a triathlon training program, your body will use a lot of carbohydrates to fuel exercise. Before getting into what this fuel source is all about, let me answer that nagging question, "If I'm not using much fat during exercise and I'm not in very good shape now, how will I ever lose weight by exercising?" The answer is in the sidebar "The Fat-Burning Zone Myth." A one-sentence summary: More calories are burned after exercise as your metabolism speeds up than during exercise, and these post-workout calories come primarily from fat due to an increase in your resting metabolic rate (discussed in Chapter 2).

Although even the fittest triathlete has a lot of calories stored as fat in his or her body—enough calories to fuel even an Ironman-distance triathlon, or several of them, in fact—none of us has a lot of carbohydrates packed away. Let's take a skinny male triathlete who weighs 150 pounds and has 7 percent body fat. That's a little more than 10 pounds of fat. Each pound of fat is about 3,500 calories, so our lean friend theoretically has more than 35,000 calories available just from his fat. If it were possible for him to use only fat during his Ironman race, and he burns 700 calories per hour for the 10 hours it takes him to finish, he could do

The Fat-Burning Zone Myth

For years we have been told that there is a low-intensity, fat-burning zone, and that if we exercise at that level of intensity we'll lose weight faster than at any other level of intensity. This myth is so well established that it may never go away. But I'll keep trying to dispel it anyway.

It really doesn't matter how much fat you burn during exercise. More importantly, it matters how much is burned during recovery following exercise. Extensive research backs this up. For example, one study examined the relative benefits of low- and high-intensity exercise for fat loss (Tremblay et al. 1994). In the low-intensity group of subjects, eight men and nine women pedaled four or five times each week for 20 weeks. Their intensity, based on heart rate, could be described as easy to moderate—the "fat-burning zone." The high-intensity group, made up of five men and five women, pedaled the same number of days each week, but for only 15 weeks. Their sessions lasted just long enough to include a warm-up, intervals, and a cooldown. The intervals were 15–90 seconds long and done at a very high level of effort, with long recoveries between the intervals.

The low-intensity group used more than twice as many calories during each of their exercise sessions as the high-intensity group. Yet when it came time to check body fatness with calipers, the high-intensity pedalers had lost significantly more fat. The reason for this is that following the more intense exercise sessions, their metabolism stayed high for much longer than that of the moderate pedalers. Other research has shown that one intense workout can increase a person's resting metabolic rate for up to 36 hours. So more total fat is burned after high-intensity exercise, with most of it melting off during rest. The scientists confirmed what was happening by measuring the enzymes that burn fat. They were greatly elevated in the high-intensity subjects, but there was no change in the low-intensity folks.

The bottom line? Forget about the so-called fat-burning zone during exercise. Such thinking is counterproductive. Going slow for a long time won't make you svelte.

the race five times nonstop without running out of energy—and without refueling.

This will never happen, because of the other fuel—carbohydrates. We don't have very much onboard. Carbohydrates are stored in the liver and in all the muscles throughout the body as "glycogen." Carbohydrates in the blood are called "glucose." You have perhaps 1,500–2,000 calories in this tank, depending on your size and fitness level. Big people and aerobically fit athletes store more of this precious commodity.

While 1,500–2,000 calories may sound like a lot, it really isn't. If our skinny triathlete used only carbohydrates to fuel his exercise, he would last for little more than two hours. That's hardly enough to finish an Ironman. To make matters worse for him, all the carbohydrates are not available, since not every muscle is used when, for example, he is riding his bike. The glycogen in his arms, upper back, face, and other body parts is not being called on to provide fuel for the body even though a lot is needed by the legs. The carbohydrates stored in the arm muscles simply refuse to make the pilgrimage to the legs to provide fuel. So our friend is forced to rely on the carbohydrates stored in just his leg muscles, unless he takes in some carbohydrates during the race. (More on this later.)

In the real world the body never relies on just one fuel source; it is always using some mix of both. When you are going slow and easy, fat is the primary fuel, but some amount of carbohydrates is still contributing calories. (Again, be sure to read "The Fat-Burning Zone Myth" sidebar.) As you start exercising faster and harder, the body shifts to more reliance on carbohydrates, although some fat is still being used.

Table 3.2 shows what your body is relying on for fuel when you exercise at different intensities.

The body simply cannot operate on only one fuel. If you start to run low on one of them—carbohydrates, obviously—you simply can't go on. This is referred to as "bonking." The way to prevent the bonk is to take in carbohydrates both before and during exercise. We've already looked at fueling before exercise, so now let's examine what to take in while you're working out.

Table 3.2 Fuel Sources at Different Workout Intensities

INTENSITY	% CARBOHYDRATES/FAT
Zone 1—very easy	about 50/50
Zone 2—easy	about 60/40
Zone 3—moderately hard	about 70/30
Zone 4—hard	about 80/20
Zone 5—very hard	about 90/10

If before your workout you consume some food, sports drink, or gel with water, and your workout lasts less than an hour, as most will in the training plan in Chapter 9, all you need to take in during the exercise session is water. It's okay to use a sports drink in this situation, but it is not necessary. (By the way, if you are trying to reduce body fat, consuming the unneeded sugar in a sports drink is not going to help.) For longer workouts or for those that start early in the morning after an overnight fast, it's a good idea to choose a product designed for use during exercise. Avoid fruit juice, as the fructose in it moves to the muscles very slowly. It could also upset your stomach during exercise. That's common for a lot of people. Also, don't drink only plain water if your workout will take more than an hour—supplement with a sports drink.

You only need a few ounces of sports drink per hour while exercising, depending on your size, how hard you are working, the weather, and most importantly, your thirst. On hot or humid days when you are going fast and hard you will need more than on cooler days with easy workouts. Your thirst will tell you so. Learn to pay attention to—and to satisfy—your thirst during workouts and you will not dehydrate. The more difficult question to answer is how you will get enough calories in if you use thirst as a guide for drinking a sports drink. Experimentation during longer workouts (i.e., those lasting more than an hour) is the best way to find out. You may need to separate fluids from calories during exercise if you don't need to drink much. In that case gels may be the better choice. Table 3.3 provides a summary of how to use sports nutrition products to

Table 3.3 How to Refuel During Exercise

EXERCISE DURATION	WATER	SPORTS DRINK	GELS	BARS/ BLOCKS
Under 1 hour with pre-workout fuel	x			
Under 1 hour with no pre-workout fuel	x	x		
1–4 hours	x	x	x	x
4 or more hours	x	x	x	x

refuel during exercise. These products include various combinations of sugars, protein, fat, electrolytes, caffeine, vitamins, minerals, and other scientific-sounding ingredients. It gets confusing, so to help clear the haze, here's a short primer.

Sports Nutrition Products

In the last three decades there has been a profound revolution in sports nutrition. It all started in the 1960s with a sports drink developed at the University of Florida—Gatorade. The field has expanded well beyond drinks consumed during exercise, and there are now more products on the market than can be sampled in a four-hour workout, including carbohydrate-loading drinks, recovery drinks, sports bars, and energy gels.

SPORTS DRINKS

Researchers at the University of Florida launched this product category in 1965 when they created a drink for the school's football team, which they later named Gatorade after the school's mascot. Before Gatorade, athletes were discouraged from drinking any fluids at all during exercise, including water. Today this is unthinkable. Sports drinks today always include a sugar and usually have some amount of sodium. Fluid and sugar are the most critical components of any sports drink. There typically are other ingredients as well, including additional minerals (e.g., potassium, magnesium, and calcium), caffeine, protein, fat, amino acids, and vitamins. The other ingredients may or may not be beneficial. The research is not overwhelming for any of them, including sodium. Sports drinks, or some sort of sugar-and-fluid source, are critical for long and highly intense workouts and races. For workouts lasting less than an hour water will do just fine.

SPORTS BARS

In the 1980s, PowerBar launched a new category of sports nutritionals—sports bars. Although they look much like candy bars, the primary ingredient is usually a sugar-based carbohydrate, and all contain some fat and protein. Most have less than 3 grams of fat, although some have twice that amount. Others are relatively high in protein. Many sports bar companies make more than one type of bar, so read the label carefully to ensure you get what you want. Examples are PowerBar, Clif Bar, and Balance Bar.

Bars can be used in low-intensity exercise lasting longer than about 90 minutes, but two hours or longer is probably best when using bars, as they are processed more slowly than sports drinks. The major limiter for these products is their absorption rate. You must drink 8–16 ounces

Recovery Smoothie

This simple recipe makes a drink of about 250–300 calories.

   8–12 oz. fruit juice of your choice

   1 serving fruit (such as a banana or frozen berries)

   1–2 pinches salt

   1–2 teaspoons protein powder

   1–2 handfuls ice

Puree the ingredients in a blender. For longer and harder workouts, add 1 tablespoon of sugar, which is about 50 calories.

of fluid with every bar eaten, and it still may take several minutes for its fuel to get to your working muscles.

GELS

Energy gels, which entered the sports nutrition field in the mid-1990s, are gooey, honey-like liquids that come in ketchup-sized pouches to be torn open and sucked out. They offer the convenience of a small package and a high energy yield—about 100 calories per packet. In this category are PowerBar Gel, Accel Gel, Carb BOOM!, GU, Hammer Gel, Lava Gel, and Clif Shot. During exercise lasting one to four hours, take one gel packet every 30 minutes. For races or workouts lasting about four hours or more, you're likely to need three or even four packets an hour depending on your body size. Be sure to drink 8–10 ounces of water with each packet.

Be careful to take in enough water when using sports bars and gels. If you don't, your gut will pull fluid from your blood to help in the digestive process. This can contribute to dehydration.

BLOCKS

Blocks are the most recent sports nutrition product. These are gummy-bear-like, solid cubes of sugar containing ingredients similar to all the others. It seems that some people love these and others hate them. You'll have to try them yourself to see in which camp you fall.

As with sports bars, blocks are probably best for long events lasting three to four hours or more, since they dissolve somewhat slowly in the gut. They should be chased with several large gulps of water to aid digestion.

REFUELING AFTER EXERCISE

Immediately after exercise your body has two primary needs—water and carbohydrates. To a lesser extent it also needs essential amino acids. For workouts that are long, highly intense, and/or hot, you'll need more of all these. The sooner you consume them after stopping, the sooner you will be ready for the next workout. I tell the athletes I coach that refueling is their highest priority right after exercise. Within the first 30 minutes after training, before stretching, taking a shower, or anything else, they should start refueling. At this time the body is better primed to accept and restock carbohydrates in the muscles and the liver than at any other time in the day.

Following a long or difficult workout or race, use something a bit more potent than a sports drink, gel, bar, or blocks. You can purchase commercial recovery drinks, but making them in your own kitchen is more cost-effective. See my recipe for a fruit smoothie that can be used after workouts lasting more than one hour. For easy workouts lasting less than an hour, fruit juice alone or mixed with a little sports drink on the strong side is a good choice.

When shopping for protein powder, look first for egg protein. This may be hard to find, so the next best option is egg and whey protein or whey alone. Third best is soy powder. Avoid vegetable protein powder, as it is missing several essential amino acids needed for recovery.

An hour or so following a one-hour or longer workout, and after previously taking in a recovery drink, it's time to move on to regular food. If you're an experienced swimmer, biker, or runner, and you complete a much longer and harder workout, you may well need another recovery drink and more time to recover before sitting down to a meal. In this case, figure that for every minute of exercise beyond one hour you will spend one minute in this short-term recovery phase taking in a recovery drink and starchy foods such as potatoes, cereal, bread, bagels, rice, pasta, or corn. These foods are rich in glucose, a form of sugar that the body uses to quickly replace its workout-depleted stores of carbohydrates.

But if you're not doing difficult workouts longer than an hour, use only fruit juice or a slightly stronger mixture of a sports drink in the first 30 minutes after stopping and then, later on, have a meal of real food. Don't rely on recovery foods, sports bars, gels, or energy drinks beyond this point in your day. Not only will they add unwanted body weight, but they are low in the micronutrients—the vitamins and minerals—necessary for good health and fitness.

EATING DURING THE REST OF THE DAY

Up to this point the emphasis of before, during, and after exercise nutrition has been on carbohydrates, especially from sugar-rich sources such as sports drinks, gels, bars, blocks, and also starchy foods. The purpose of all this sugar is to keep your muscle and liver glycogen stores up so that you don't run out of fuel. If you've done a good job, you don't need to be as concerned with quick-acting forms of carbohydrates during the rest of the day.

After your initial recovery from exercise, the emphasis shifts to eating foods that are rich in all the essential nutrients. This includes essential amino acids from protein-rich foods, carbohydrates with lots of vitamins and minerals, and healthy fats.

Essential Amino Acids

Amino acids make up protein, which is found in almost all foods but especially in animal products such as fish, poultry, red meat, and eggs. My experience in working with athletes for more than three decades is that they tend to eat too little protein because they focus their diets on sugar and starch. That's too bad, because the amino acids in protein are necessary for the growth, repair, and maintenance of your muscles, immune system, and other cells. I've come to realize that athletes who eat too little protein will recover slowly after workouts, are easily injured, and never achieve their full potential in triathlons. You can't skimp on protein if you want to get in shape.

Scientists have identified 20 amino acids necessary for human development. Eight of these are essential amino acids because your adult body can't make them. Animal foods are rich in these essentials, while plant foods are each lacking in some of them. But it's possible to combine plant foods to prepare a meal that has all the essential amino acids. A common way some vegetarians do this is to mix beans and grains together (e.g., beans and rice or peanut butter and bread). The downside is that you have to eat a lot more vegetable food, including a lot of starch, to get the same amount of essential amino acids that are in animal foods. For example, a 2-ounce serving of turkey breast has about 7 grams of essential amino acids and 100 calories. To get the same amount from a meal

Table 3.4 Protein and Essential Amino Acids in Common Foods

	FOOD (100-KCAL SERVING)	PROTEIN (GRAMS)	ESSENTIAL AMINO ACID (GRAMS)
ANIMAL	Cod (3.4 oz.)	22	8.7
	Shrimp (3.6 oz.)	21	8.2
	Lobster (3.6 oz.)	21	8.1
	Halibut (2.5 oz.)	19	7.5
	Chicken (2 oz.)	18	6.8
	Turkey breast (2 oz.)	17	6.9
	Tuna (1.9 oz.)	16	6.3
	Tenderloin steak (1.75 oz.)	14	5.1
	Egg, whole (1.25 oz.)	7.7	3.4
LEGUMES	Tofu (½ cup)	10	3.6
	Kidney beans (½ cup)	7	2.8
	Navy beans (⅓ cup)	6	1.9
	Red beans (½ cup)	5	2.5
	Peanut butter (1 tbsp.)	4.6	1.4
GRAINS	Bagel (½ bagel)	3.8	1.1
	Corn (¾ cup)	3.7	1.4
	Whole wheat bread (1½ slices)	3	0.8
	Brown rice (½ cup)	2.1	0.7

of red beans and rice, you'd have to eat 1½ cups of rice and a cup of beans at a total of 500 calories. That's a lot of beans and rice. And there are five times as many calories in the beans and rice as in the turkey.

Unless you need to gain a lot of weight (and really like beans!), the surest way to provide your body with the building supplies needed to get into shape is to eat animal products. This doesn't mean you should cut out vegetables, however, as they are rich in vitamins and minerals. Table 3.4 lists the protein and the essential amino acid content in several animal foods along with commonly combined legumes and grains in 100-calorie serving sizes.

Vitamins and Minerals

When most people talk about carbohydrates they mean starchy foods such as cereal, bread, bagels, rice, corn, and potatoes. While these are indeed carbohydrate-based foods, they make up only one part of this food category. We tend to forget that fruits and vegetables are also in the carbohydrate group. More of these foods, especially vegetables, are needed in meals after the 30-minute recovery period following the day's last workout, because veggies have more vitamins and minerals than any other foods you could eat.

Because vitamins and minerals are necessary to promote growth and to maintain health, if your diet is deficient in them you run the risk of a slow response to training and perhaps even disease. People who eat a lot of food every day and never exercise don't have to worry about this, but if you are watching your calories and exercising a lot, the risk is greater.

Vegetables in general have far more vitamins and minerals than any other food group. Spinach has 65 percent more calcium per calorie than milk; broccoli, rhubarb, turnip greens, and watercress also have more calcium per calorie than milk. Other minerals necessary for strenuous exercise, such as iron, magnesium, phosphorus, potassium, and zinc, are also found in great quantities in vegetables. In addition, veggies are loaded with the exercise-critical B vitamins and antioxidants such as vitamins E and C. As a group, vegetables have nearly twice as much vitamins and minerals as most other food groups. Table 3.5 illustrates this. It may look complex, so I'll explain it.

Listed across the top of Table 3.5 are the food categories. Included in each category are the most commonly eaten foods in the U.S. diet: 8 whole grains, whole milk, 20 fruits, 18 vegetables, 20 types of seafood, 4 lean meats, and 10 seeds and nuts. Down the left side are the 13 vitamins and minerals most frequently lacking or deficient in the U.S. diet. The average vitamin and mineral nutrient values for each of these foods are also included, and the values for the nutrients are compared and ranked (7 = *highest average value*; 1 = *lowest average value*). The small superscript number shows the rankings for each vitamin and mineral within a food category.

Across the bottom of the table is a sum of the superscript rankings by category. The most nutritious food group, in other words the one with

Table 3.5 Nutrient Values for Various Food Groups (100-kcal serving)

MICRONUTRIENT	WHOLE GRAINS	WHOLE MILK	FRUITS
Calcium (mg)	7.6^2	**194.3**^{7}	43.0^4
Folate (µg)	10.3^4	8.1^2	25.0^6
Iron (mg)	0.90^4	0.08^1	0.69^2
Magnesium (mg)	32.6^4	21.9^2	24.6^3
Phosphorus (mg)	90^3	152^5	33^1
Vitamin A (RE)	2^2	50^5	94^6
Vitamin B1 (mg)	0.12^5	0.06^1	0.11^3
Vitamin B2 (mg)	0.05^2	0.26^6	0.09^3
Vitamin B3 (mg)	1.12^4	0.14^1	0.89^3
Vitamin B6 (mg)	0.09^3	0.07^1	0.20^5
Vitamin B12 (µg)	0	0.58^5	0
Vitamin C (mg)	1.53^3	74.2^5	**221.3**^{7}
Zinc (mg)	0.67^4	0.62^3	0.25^1
Sum rank score	44	44	48

Note: Superscripts represent each micronutrient's relative ranking from 1 (*lowest average value*) to 7 (*highest average value*) relative to the other food groups. The highest value for each food group is in boldface type.

the most vitamins and minerals, is, hands-down, vegetables. Next is seafood followed by lean meats. Bringing up the rear are whole grains, milk, and seeds and nuts.

So as you can see, the food groups with the least vitamins and minerals are whole grains, dairy, and seeds and nuts. This doesn't mean you should never eat these foods. But if you are exercising strenuously and watching your calories, you want to eat mostly nutrient-dense foods. That means lots of veggies.

Healthy Fats

We've been taught that fat is bad for our health and told to restrict it in our diets. That's a bit like throwing the baby out with the bathwater. The problem isn't the amount of fat in your diet but rather the type of fat. Fat is necessary for immune system health and adds a pleasing flavor and

VEGETABLES	SEAFOOD	LEAN MEATS	SEEDS, NUTS
116.8[6]	43.1[5]	6.1[1]	17.5[3]
208.3[7]	10.8[3]	3.8[1]	11.0[5]
2.59[7]	2.07[6]	1.10[5]	0.86[3]
54.5[7]	36.1[6]	18.0[1]	35.8[5]
157[6]	219[7]	151[4]	80[2]
687[7]	32[4]	1[1]	2[3]
0.26[7]	0.08[2]	0.18[6]	0.12[4]
0.33[7]	0.09[4]	0.14[5]	0.04[1]
2.73[5]	3.19[6]	4.73[7]	0.35[2]
0.42[7]	0.19[4]	0.32[6]	0.08[2]
0.63[6]	7.42[7]	0.63[6]	0.63[6]
93.6[6]	1.9[4]	0.1[1]	0.4[2]
1.04[5]	7.6[7]	1.9[6]	0.6[2]
81	65	50	38

Source: Adapted with permission from Loren Cordain and Joe Friel, The Paleo Diet for Athletes, 2nd ed. (New York: Rodale Books, 2012).

Energizing Exercise

Fat and carbohydrate are the body's main fuel sources. Understanding the role each plays in exercise will help you decide how to train to achieve certain benefits, and how to recover from workouts.

Fat is the major fuel for all endurance exercise. "Endurance" means continuous exercise lasting longer than about two minutes. Even the skinniest athlete has several hours of energy stored in his or her body as fat.

Carbohydrates are stored as either "glycogen" in the muscles and liver or "glucose" in the blood. Glycogen makes up most of this energy source, but it is quite limited. A well-conditioned athlete may have enough glycogen for two to three hours of intense exercise. When glycogen runs low, exercise must slow down, regardless of how much fat is available. This is one reason why it is so important to take in carbohydrates during workouts lasting longer than about an hour.

It may sound as if the body switches from one energy source to another. That's not the case. There is considerable overlap among the fuels used in a workout, with the percentages fluctuating in relation to intensity, warm-up, and fitness level.

As endurance exercise begins, the first few seconds are fueled primarily by creatine phosphate as the fat- and glycogen-processing mechanisms kick in. In the next several minutes—perhaps 10 to 30—glycogen supplies much of the energy, with fat slowly increasing its contribution, if the workout is a steady effort. Eventually, fat becomes the predominant fuel source for long and slow exercise, with glycogen adding most of the balance.

This doesn't mean that slow exercise is the best way to burn fat; the total energy expenditure during light activity is low when compared with fast and intense workouts. Although the percentage of fat burned in intense exercise—such as intervals—is smaller, the total energy used is larger, potentially producing a greater amount of total fat use.

texture to food. The right types of fat even help reduce your likelihood of injury from exercise while speeding your healing should you still have a tendon or muscle flare-up. If you cut out the "good" fats in your diet, you simply won't train as well. You just need to be aware of and control how much you eat when it comes to the three "bad" fats—saturated fat, trans fat, and polyunsaturated omega-6 oil. These fats have been shown to contribute to health problems such as heart disease, skin cancer, diabetes, and asthma. It doesn't matter if you are a triathlete or a couch spud; these fats just aren't good for anyone.

These bad fats are found in such food sources as feedlot-raised and factory-farmed animals, snack foods, packaged meals, margarine, and whole-fat dairy products, and in such ubiquitous products as peanut butter, bread, bagels, salad dressing, and even some frozen vegetables. When you shop, read the labels carefully and avoid those products listing saturated fat and partially hydrogenated fat and those made with vegetable oils such as soybean, peanut, cottonseed, safflower, sunflower, sesame, and corn. You'll find this cuts out a lot of foods. But you'll quickly become familiar with the best packaged foods.

The fats you should get more of in your diet are monounsaturated fat and polyunsaturated omega-3 oil as these meet your daily need for fat and promote good health. These are found in nuts, especially macadamias and walnuts, avocados, olive oil, canola oil, cold-water fish (e.g., salmon, mackerel, herring, halibut, cod, and tuna), leafy green vegetables, and flaxseed oil. Not only will you be healthier for eating these good fats, but you'll also improve your aerobic fitness, recover from exercise faster, and may even reduce post-exercise soreness. I advise the athletes I coach to supplement their diets with fish oil capsules because it is difficult to get enough omega-3 oil from our modern diet. In fact, this and vitamin D taken in the winter months are the only supplements I recommend you take. A healthy diet, as described with a focus on veggies, seafood, lean meats, and good fats, as listed in Table 3.6, will give you all the other vitamins and minerals needed.

Table 3.6 Fats: The Good, the Okay, the Bad, and the Ugly

MONOUNSATURATED AND POLYUNSATURATED OMEGA-3 FAT *Include some of these good fats in daily meals and snacks.*

Macadamia nuts	Herring
Walnuts	Halibut
Avocados	Cod
Canola oil	Tuna
Olive oil	Leafy green vegetables
Salmon	Flaxseed oil
Mackerel	Nut butters

POLYUNSATURATED OMEGA-6 FAT *It's okay to include some in your diet, but avoid eating a lot of these fats, especially in packaged foods.*

Soybean oil	Corn oil
Peanut oil	Sunflower seeds and oil
Cottonseed oil	Sesame seeds and oil
Safflower oil	Pumpkin seeds and oil

SATURATED FAT *Strictly limit your intake of bad fats.*

Fatty cuts of meat (beef, lamb, pork)	Cheese
Chicken with skin	Ice cream
Whole milk and cream	Lard
Butter	

TRANS FAT *Avoid ugly foods that say "partially hydrogenated" on the label.*

Stick margarine	Most packaged snack foods (microwave popcorn, potato chips)
Most commercial pastries (doughnuts, cookies, cakes, etc.)	Vegetable shortening
Some packaged grains (bread, bagel, cereal, crackers)	Most fast foods
Some salad dressings	Most fried foods (french fries, fried chicken, chicken nuggets, breaded fish)
Some commercial soups	Some peanut butters
Candy bars	

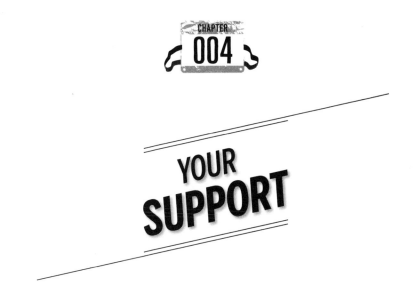

CHAPTER 004

YOUR SUPPORT

W ith all this talk about *your diet*, *your lifestyle*, and *your training plan*, I hope I haven't led you to believe that to become a triathlete you will have to live like a hermit, coming out of your cave only to swim, bike, and run. It's true that triathlon is ultimately an individual sport requiring self-sufficiency, but it doesn't have to be a lonely sport. You'll find that triathletes, as a whole, are fun, gregarious people who love to be with others. And if you want to succeed in the sport, you will certainly need the help of others—your supporters.

EMOTIONAL SUPPORT

On the whole, training for a triathlon brings great pleasure. Motivation comes easily when you realize that your fitness and endurance are improving as your waistline is trimming. But there will be times when none of this seems to be happening. You may feel weary and as if you have too many responsibilities to manage. At these times you need the encouragement of your family and friends to keep going. Without their support, you're likely to fall off the wagon.

Family

Your spouse is your most important supporter. I once coached a runner who wanted to qualify for the Boston Marathon and had a chance, although he was going to have to run his best race ever to do it. His wife, however, thought that running was just plain dumb. She gave him a hard time whenever he went out to run. So he got in the habit of getting out of bed several hours early on Saturdays so he could get his long run done and be back by the time his wife woke up. Whenever possible he hid his running from her. He had no support at home for his goal. Needless to say, he did not qualify despite his hard work.

The most supportive spouses are often those who also are physically active. It's easier for them to empathize with a partner who is aspiring to be more athletic. But I also know many spouses who are 100 percent supportive even though they never swim, bike, or run. You can foster such support by sharing in your spouse's dreams and aspirations. Being honestly enthusiastic about your partner's activities is the starting point. Be sure to make him or her a part of your team by sharing your experiences and achievements and by asking for help whenever you need it. You can also wrap a vacation around a triathlon so the whole family has something to look forward to.

Friends

There's no getting around it—triathletes are unusual people. We carefully avoid unhealthy food, exercise before and after work, enjoy sweating, talk incessantly about our last workout, and ogle fast bikes the way a starving man looks at food. Only other triathletes can fully understand such strange behavior. Yet there are nontriathletes who continue to hang out with us happily and even feign an interest in our obsession. We call these people *friends*. We need lots of them if we're to make it in triathlon. They may not always understand what we are talking about, but they always care and are there when we need them. Such people are truly good friends whose support we must carefully nurture. So don't lay it all on them at once—and realize that they may have something of interest in their lives also. Support works both ways. We must be willing to go the extra mile for friends who support us. This may occasionally mean making the ultimate sacrifice—missing a workout. I think it's safe to say that what we get out of our friendships will be in direct proportion to how much we give.

TRAINING SUPPORT

Triathlon can be a lonely sport. It's really nice to occasionally have someone along for a workout. A steady diet of solo exercise can be mind-numbing, or worse—it can contribute to a loss of motivation. It's a rare person who can do every workout alone and remain enthusiastic. A training partner, or better yet, a group is the best therapy for boredom and low motivation.

Clubs

Many larger cities and even some small ones have triathlon clubs. These groups often offer weekly workouts in one or more of the three disciplines and publish newsletters with information of local interest. Some clubs host periodic meetings with prominent guest speakers and even have coaches who can help you grow as a triathlete. Check with USA Triathlon, the governing body of the sport in the United States, to find out if there's a triathlon club in your area. If there isn't a club near you, consider starting one. USA Triathlon can help you with this, too.

Training Partners

If there just aren't any clubs in your area, finding another triathlete of your ability will do wonders for your motivation. You will discover that it's easier to get out of bed in the morning or go for an after-work training session if you know your training partner will be there, too. In the winter months, getting together with a training partner for an indoor bike-trainer ride or a side-by-side treadmill run will boost not only the quality but also the enjoyment of such workouts.

Chances are good that your local triathlon or running shop is frequented by triathletes. Some shops have bulletin boards to facilitate the search for a training partner or they might host weekly group workouts. If you belong to a gym, you might find similar opportunities there. Social networking sites are yet another ticket to finding a training partner with similar goals.

TECHNICAL SUPPORT

Getting in shape, dealing with or preventing injuries, and buying and maintaining the right equipment are all huge tasks. Each is so complex that it is impossible to keep up with even the most basic technical information. Specialists are the answer.

Medical Examinations

When I start coaching an athlete, one of the first things I do is to have him or her see a physical therapist for a thorough orthopedic exam. I want to know where the weak links are and what we can do to prevent injury. The most common problems found, even in otherwise seemingly sound athletes, are poor spinal health, unstable knees, muscle imbalances, leg-length discrepancies, flat feet, and poor posture. The therapist can suggest strength and flexibility exercises or other options to alleviate the negative consequences of such conditions. I find this to be an invaluable step to prevent injuries and optimize performance. It's money well spent when you're just starting out.

It helps if your doctor values an active lifestyle or at least understands why you do it and supports your pursuit. In the past, when a patient came in complaining of a sore knee from running, the doctor would prescribe aspirin and suggest no more such foolishness as jogging. Nowadays sports medicine is a booming business, and if your doctor doesn't know exactly how to handle your aches and pains, he or she can refer you to a sports specialist. The world of triathlon is much better because of this development in medicine.

Coaching

The field of triathlon coaching is expanding every year. What was once a hobby for a few has become a career for many. USA Triathlon now lists about two thousand certified triathlon coaches on its web site. At this site you can find a coach to help you grow as a triathlete. I recommend finding someone who lives in your area, since you are new to the sport and will need face-to-face coaching as you develop skills. Once you are skilled and have more experience, there are many more coaches available who work via the Internet. You can find coaches I have trained at www.trainingbible.com.

Coaching fees vary considerably, from free to hundreds of dollars a month. You typically get just what you pay for, so don't let price be the only determining factor. It's a good idea to interview at least three coaches before making a final selection. You'll discover that there are considerable differences in the services they offer. You also will probably find that you relate best to one of them. That's the one for you.

Besides designing and refining a training plan for you, a good coach will provide advice on equipment purchases, diet, race strategy, and motivation. In fact, just having a coach is usually good for motivation. He or she is part of your team.

Equipment

It used to be the case that sporting goods stores specializing in swim, bike, or run gear were the unchallenged center of the triathlon universe. That's where you went to buy anything needed for the sport. In recent years, mail-order and online catalogs have the playing field. In order to compete, triathlon retailers have begun offering a lot more than just equipment; they also offer information, quality bicycle repair and maintenance, and other specialized services. Good shops also make sure you buy the right stuff in a world of ever-increasing equipment complexity. Such shops become the places to go to find event flyers, to get training questions answered, or to have your bike adjusted to help an aching knee.

It behooves you to make your purchases at a local shop. The prices are not significantly higher than catalog or online costs once shipping is added on. Even if you spend a couple of dollars more, the services you get are certainly worth the small extra expense.

WHERE TO FIND MORE INFORMATION

Triathlon is one of the youngest sports in the world, having been around since only the 1970s. In the 1980s and the 1990s the number of participants and races grew steadily, but following its Olympic debut in the 2000 Sydney Games, triathlon has grown exponentially. In the United States there were about 20,000 USA Triathlon–licensed triathletes in 2000. By 2004 the number had more than doubled to 53,000. As of January 2011, USA Triathlon had 135,000 members—nearly a sevenfold rate of growth in just over 10 years. And there are perhaps that many again who participate in local triathlons without getting an annual license. Few sports have grown so fast in such a short time.

Due to triathlon's recent rapid growth, information on the sport is overwhelming. It's impossible to keep up with it all, so pick a couple of sources from the following suggestions and use them to learn more about your sport.

Online Resources

A Google search on "triathlon" will yield millions of results. Newsgroups, bulletin boards, blogs, web sites, chat rooms, online magazines, and live talks by experts abound. It isn't possible to list all of them here, but the following are a few that may prove helpful:

> *Race calendars.* Are you planning a vacation and wanting to see if there's a triathlon you could do at your destination? Or perhaps you just want to see what's available in your region. A good Internet site for this information is www.activeglobal.com. Here you can both find a race listing and complete an entry form online.

General triathlon information. Want to see what others also new to the sport are doing as they prepare for a triathlon? Go to www.trinewbies.com. For basic information on training, race reports, and firsthand experiences, go to www.hulaman.com. This is the oldest free triathlon training site on the web. Two of the largest discussion sites for triathletes on all matters related to the sport may be found at groups.google.com/group/rec.sport.triathlon and www.slowtwitch.com.

Coaching. For assistance finding a triathlon coach, go to www.trainingpeaks.com or to www.usatriathlon.org.

Training log. Store and analyze your training data on www.trainingpeaks.com. There is also a forum where you can get your triathlon questions answered by a professional coach.

Print Media

Although triathlon sites on the World Wide Web are prodigious, print media on this topic in the United States are rather limited. Two magazines dominate the national scene: *Inside Triathlon* and *Triathlete*. The same publishing group now owns both publications. *Triathlete* has been around since the early 1980s and provides extensive coverage of professional racing plus age-group coverage and plenty of training information. *Inside Triathlon* is a lifestyle magazine with more in-depth articles on the top triathletes, the technical aspects of training, and the research in sport and performance. Both magazines offer print or digital subscriptions, and can be found on the newsstand (go to triathlon.competitor.com for more information). In addition, many regional publications focus on triathlon, such as *Colorado Triathlete*, *Competitor* (which has multiple regional editions), and *Oklahoma Runner & Triathlete*. These are usually available in sporting goods stores, at health clubs, and on newsstands in their regions.

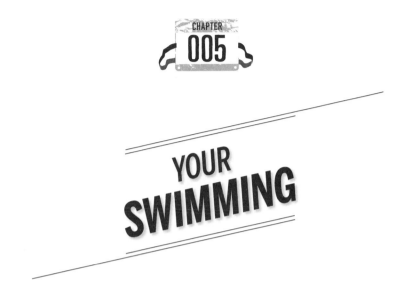

CHAPTER

005

YOUR SWIMMING

O f the three triathlon sports, you'll spend the least amount of time swimming, both during training and in the race. This is partly because the swim is so short in a sprint triathlon—usually about 400 meters (0.25 mile). If an Olympic-distance race will be your first triathlon, the 1,500-meter (0.93-mile) swim is still very short. The biking and running legs will last a lot longer, no matter which race distance you choose.

Think of the swim as a warm-up for the rest of the triathlon. If you are relatively new to swimming, your goal for the swim leg is just to finish it; it doesn't matter what your time is. You may stop several times to catch your breath. You can use several strokes besides the standard freestyle—backstroke, sidestroke, and breaststroke. That's okay; others will stop and use different strokes, too.

What we want to accomplish with your swimming at this stage of your triathlon career is not speed or great endurance but sound swimming skills—something to build on for the future. Swim training is mostly about learning good technique, whereas training for the bike and the run is mostly about building fitness. For now, good swim skills are much more important than good swim fitness.

With good technique the swimming will feel easier and you'll go faster. Remember this because it's the key to your success in the water. First-time swimmers tend to think it's the other way around and spend several weeks trying to get fit for the swim without worrying about their swim mechanics, but it doesn't work that way. You must become a more skillful swimmer first. That's how you become fast in the water.

If you are already a swimmer, this will be a breeze. You've got a great start on becoming a triathlete, because it takes months, if not years, to hone the mechanics of swimming. Just be careful not to spend most of your training time in the pool. Triathletes tend to gravitate toward what comes easiest while avoiding their weaker sports. As an accomplished swimmer, you should spend more time biking and running than those without a swim background.

FLAWED TECHNIQUE

The following are some technique flaws that are common to athletes who are just taking up swimming. Of course, here I am talking about the free-style technique, which you may know as the "crawl" stroke. Although you may choose any stroke you wish in a triathlon, the one most triathletes use, and the fastest, is freestyle. So here are some common technique errors people make when swimming using the freestyle stroke.

Face out of the Water

It's normal for mammals to keep their heads and faces out of the water when swimming, for example as a dog does. Since we don't have gills and the air is above the water, it's easy to see why this happens. Breathing is the biggest challenge in learning to swim, and it is the starting place for learning good technique. Throughout your triathlon career you'll hear athletes and swim instructors talking about how to breathe, when to breathe, and how often to breathe.

Focus on Form—Not Fitness

I can't emphasize this enough: Getting started in swimming is mostly about learning to swim properly. You can probably already swim now, meaning that you can take a few strokes without sinking and may even be able to complete one or more lengths of the pool. But most people at this stage have poor technique because they developed bad habits when they first learned to swim.

As a kid your only goal in going to the pool was to have fun with others in the water. You didn't care how much energy it took to swim after a ball or to chase your buddies. But these swimming flaws will come back to haunt you while training for your first triathlon. Poor technique uses a lot more energy than is necessary, causing you to start the bike section of the race already feeling drained.

Hips Below Shoulders

Because your face is out of the water, a line drawn from your shoulders through your hips would be slanted down, with your hips low in the water. In this position it takes more energy to move forward because you are presenting a lot of frontal area to the water. Unlike air, water is a thick, resistant medium that causes you to work hard to move through it. Once you learn to put your face in the water and breathe to the side correctly, your hips will come up, and you'll be amazed at how much easier it is to swim. It's like the difference between pushing a sheet of plywood through the water horizontally and doing it vertically.

Pushing down on the Water

In order to keep your face above the waterline, you probably push down on the water with your hands. This results in very little forward movement. Again, learning to swim and to breathe with your face in the water will go a long way toward correcting this common fault.

Kicking Too Much

Since your hands and arms aren't providing much forward movement, you end up kicking hard to go forward. In this position the kick is not very effective, so it requires a lot of effort. Once you learn to swim horizontally, with your hips at the waterline, you'll find that the kick is only needed to provide balance, not locomotion. With your body in a streamlined position, your hands and arms will do most of the work to move you forward. Keep your kick small and easy.

REINFORCING GOOD TECHNIQUE

The starting place for developing good swim technique is learning to put your face in the water and breathe to the side. Once you can do this everything else can begin to fall into place. At that point you will be working on refining technique and becoming smoother and more efficient. But for now you're tackling the essential skill—head position and breathing.

The best way to learn good swimming technique is with an instructor. I do not recommend learning to swim alone.

Work with an Instructor

The best choice for instruction is to hire a swim instructor and take a lesson once or twice a week. You will develop skills quickly with a good teacher. It's usually best not to ask a friend who is a good swimmer, as he or she likely is not a good swim teacher. Look for someone with lots of experience working with newbies.

Some instructors offer swim instruction over the Internet. They ask you to have someone use an underwater camera to make a movie of you swimming and then send it to them; an instructor analyzes it and sends you technique tips. This is much less effective than having a real, live coach watching, but if you don't have any other options, it can point you in the right direction.

Even though you have an instructor, you'll need to practice on your own to really develop your skills. Following the training schedules provided in Chapter 9 will give you that opportunity.

Swim with a Masters Class

The next best instruction option is to swim with a masters group at your health club, community pool, or YMCA. Ask around to see what's available. This is usually the least expensive route to take. Avoid joining a highly competitive, advanced group. Look for one that caters to beginners. Swim groups usually have a coach on deck who can provide feedback on your technique; ask the coach to help you whenever possible. But you are not the only person in the pool, so don't expect a lot of personal attention.

Find a Swim Camp

A third instruction option is to attend a swim camp. Triathlon and swim coaches offer camps regionally. Two good ones are Terry Laughlin (www .totalimmersion.net) and Steve Tarpinian (www.ttuniversity.com/ttu). You can read about their camp offerings online to see if there is one in your area. I also put on triathlon camps with swim instruction in North America and in Europe. Check my blog for these: www.joefrielsblog.com. While you're online, also check out a great visual aid, "Mr. Smooth," at www.swimsmooth.com.

Even with an instructor and practice, it's a good idea to learn as much as you can about swim technique. Books and videos available at retailers and online will help you see what good form looks like.

Right now your goal for swimming is not to become more fit but rather to learn to swim with good technique. As you work on your swimming skills your fitness will improve without a lot of hard work. In fact, overworking during a swim workout at this stage of your trainning is likely to cause your form to break down and reinforce your old flaws. Remember: form—not fitness!

WHERE TO SWIM

For beginners I recommend swimming in a public pool, such as at your health club, city facility, or YMCA. Even if you have a pool in your backyard you'll find that you improve faster with others around. In part, this is because you will learn from watching others who have mastered the techniques. Having others around also makes swimming safer.

At this stage in your budding triathlon career, open-water swimming, such as in lakes or the ocean, is best done infrequently. Not only is open water inherently risky, but such swimming also makes it more difficult to develop good technique. A controlled pool environment with calm water, a black line to follow, and lane ropes to keep you corralled provides just enough structure to keep you focused on form. There are too many variables in open water to allow you to concentrate on stroke mechanics. If, however, your race will be done in a lake or in the ocean, then you need to get in at least two open-water swims. These are best done in the last four weeks before your race.

The first skill to learn in open-water swimming is sighting on fixed objects so that you swim a straight line. The rougher the water, the more challenging this is. Every fifth stroke or so, raise your head to be sure your progress relative to the landmark is correct. This landmark may be a tall building, a tree, a pier, or something similar. In the race it may be a large buoy. It's best to have several such objects you can use for navigating during your swim.

A word of caution: Never swim alone in open water. Always have at least one partner who stays close. This is something I require even with the pro triathletes I coach.

Pool Etiquette

Most of your swimming will be done in a pool. Understanding and following pool etiquette are necessary to make swimming safe and enjoyable for everyone. Space is limited in a lap pool. The lanes are narrow and there may be a lot of swimmers trying to use them. Unwritten pool etiquette rules help the pool handle lots of people. Following are the more common rules; if there is any confusion about the specific rules where you are swimming, check with a lifeguard.

Rule 1: Choose an appropriate lane. If the pool is busy, there may be signs at the lanes specifying pace. The signs could be as simple as "Fast," "Medium," and "Slow," or they might be designated by swim pace, such as 1:30 per 100 yards for one lane and 1:45 per 100 yards in the next lane. If there aren't any designations, assess which lane has swimmers in it who are going about your pace. If there are open lanes without reserved signs or something similar, feel free to take any one of them.

Rule 2: Enter the water safely. Don't dive in. Not only is it unsafe, it's also rude. Lower yourself into the water feet first or go down a ladder. If there is someone else in the lane, before you start, stand to the side until you are certain you have been seen. Give the other person plenty of time to establish a gap and then begin swimming.

Rule 3: Share the lane. If you're entering a lane that has one other swimmer in it, ask if he or she wants to split the lane, each keeping to a side, or swim a circle, staying to the right. The first person in the lane "owns" it, so don't assume without asking. If you're the third to enter the lane and there are two already splitting it, stand to the side and wait for an opportunity to ask if you can share their lane and all swim in a circle. Circle swimming is almost always done counterclockwise by staying as close as possible to the lane rope on the right, with the black line on the bottom of the pool serving as a lane divider. But I've seen some places where they swim clockwise. Ask before starting.

Rule 4: Pass politely. If someone wants to pass you in the pool when swimming circles, he or she will touch you on the foot. Do not stop—continue swimming, but stay close to the lane rope in case he or she decides to pass now. If your foot has been tapped but the other swimmer doesn't pass you at the next wall, pause in the corner and let the faster swimmer make the turn before you start swimming again. If you are the "passer," touch the other person's foot only once. Repeated touching is annoying.

Rule 5: Stay out of the way when resting. It's okay to stop and take a breather, but stop only at a wall, and squeeze into a corner of the lane next to the rope. If you're going to pause for several minutes, get out of the pool.

Rule 6: Ask before using pool equipment. Most pools have buoys, kickboards, and other swim aids available for use. Before using one of these, ask a lifeguard for permission. If there is equipment at the end of a lane that has swimmers in it, assume someone else is using it.

Conquering the Fear of Open Water

Back in 1985 a friend of mine decided to do his first open-water triathlon. It was an Olympic-distance race with a 1,500-meter (0.93-mile) swim in a small lake. The race was in Wyoming in the spring, so the water was cold, and we all wore wet suits. Dave was a good pool swimmer who usually swam about the same pace as I did in pool workouts. When the race started, Dave was right next to me, but he quickly disappeared. After the race I found him sitting quietly in my car in the parking area. He told me that he had panicked in the first few minutes of the swim and headed straight back to the shore. He was devastated. It looked like the end of his new triathlon lifestyle, and all because of a great fear of open water.

Being a fighter, Dave decided not to throw in the towel but instead embarked on a mission to overcome his fear of open water. It took the better part of a year to accomplish this. During that time he swam in open water whenever he could find someone to go with him. He started by staying close to the shoreline, where he could easily stand up whenever he wanted. Over time he gradually moved away from the shore and learned to navigate using landmarks. He went on to be an excellent triathlete and even qualified for the Hawaii Ironman Triathlon World Championship.

Dave's story is a good example of why you should be respectful of and cautious in open water. Never take it for granted, but also don't accept fear as a normal condition. Imagining all the things that *could* go wrong only fuels fear.

When you are ready, get started in open-water swimming incrementally. Just as Dave did, stay close to the shore as you develop skills and attitudes. Venture farther out only when you're ready. Always swim with a buddy in open water—never alone, even if you're hugging the shoreline. It will take time, but you can overcome your fear of the water.

SWIMMING EQUIPMENT

You don't need much gear to get started in swimming, and the stuff you do need is not overly expensive.

Swimsuit

Obviously you need a swimsuit, and you may already have one. Some men wear a swimmer's Lycra brief-cut suit, but a tight-fitting, mid-thigh-length Lycra suit is also popular at triathlons and in pools. One nice feature of this type of longer short is that you can swim, bike, and run in it. Most styles feature a small crotch pad for cycling; however, padded swimsuits are best used only during the race, not in swim training.

Men may also wear a loose-fitting swimsuit like the one you wear when you go to the beach. You will see plenty of these in your first triathlon and at the pool. The problem with baggy swimsuits is that they slow you down because of the drag they create in the water (and later on the bike), and this drag makes learning good swim technique a bit more difficult.

I understand men's reluctance to wear formfitting Lycra in public; it definitely takes some getting used to. For now, as you get started swimming, a baggy suit will do, but observe what others at the pool are wearing, especially triathletes. Then when you feel ready, shop around for a mid-thigh-length swimsuit. Many men wear a loose-fitting pair of shorts, such as running shorts, over their Lycra swimsuit as they go to and from the locker room at the pool, taking them off just before they get in the water.

For women the traditional one-piece Lycra swimsuit is common at the pool and at triathlons. In the race you will see some women in one-piece Lycra "skinsuits." These are sleeveless, round-neck tops fastened to a thigh-length, form-fitting short with a small crotch pad for biking. Another option for the race is a separate top and bottom made like the skinsuit. Some women wear briefer shorts and tops to reduce drag in the water. As a newbie there is no reason for you to be concerned with going really fast. The standard one-piece Lycra swimsuit that you probably already have will work fine for the race and the pool. After the swim in the triathlon you can always pull on a pair of bike shorts. Many women triathletes do.

In Chapter 10 I tell you more about what to wear in your first triathlon, so here we're just concerned with what to wear at the pool. If you have to buy something, men's swimsuits run about $30–$50. Women's swimwear costs a little more, about $50–$75. One-piece skinsuits start at about $90. Separate tops and bottoms cost in the neighborhood of $40–$60 each.

Goggles

Finding the right pair of goggles can be tricky. A waterproof fit and comfort are your main concerns. You won't really be able to tell if the goggles are right until you give them a try during a swim, but to get an idea at the store, you can place the goggles on your face without putting the strap around your head. If the goggles are waterproof, you should be able to push the eyepieces against your face and feel the suction hold them in place for a couple of seconds. If they won't stay in place even for a second, then they aren't right for you. Once you've narrowed down the selection, try the finalists on with the strap around your head to see if they feel comfortable. There should be no pressure on the bridge of your nose, and they should feel as if they would stay in place even if someone bumped against you while swimming.

Two basic types of goggles are used in triathlon: the two-piece type, with separate eye lenses connected by a soft, flexible nosepiece (typically used in training), and the one-piece kind, similar to what scuba divers wear, only smaller (sometimes preferred for open-water swimming). Expect to pay anywhere from $10 to $75.

It's a good idea to have a spare pair of swim goggles for the triathlon—just in case. But don't buy these until you are certain of the best type for your face.

Swim Cap and Other Items

Most swimmers use a swim cap for training. Once you get past your first few races, you'll have lots to choose from since each race will issue a colored swim cap depending on your wave. Swim caps are perfectly practical and affordable—making you more efficient in the water and protecting your hair from chlorine damage at the same time.

Depending on your personal preference, you may also want to get a nose clip and earplugs. These can be picked up inexpensively in a general sporting goods store or at a swim specialty shop.

There are lots of other swim aids used in the pool, such as fins, kickboards, pull buoys, and other learning tools. The pool you swim at is likely to have most of these on hand, so there is no reason to buy them now. Later on you may want to consider something along this line to work on technique.

—

Notice that I didn't mention buying a wet suit. If you follow triathlon, you may be aware that in many races wet suits are worn in the swim because the open water is often cold. As mentioned earlier, if your first triathlon will be a sprint distance, then look for a pool swim. But if you are doing an Olympic-distance race, then open water is almost a certainty. In Chapter 11 I will tell you how to go about choosing a race. Should you decide to do a triathlon with a cold, open-water swim, I recommend renting a wet suit at a triathlon, swim, bike, or run store. If you go this route be sure to reserve it weeks in advance or others may beat you to it. Later, once the triathlon bug has bitten you, you can look into buying your own wet suit. This is a very technical purchase, so having more experience is helpful.

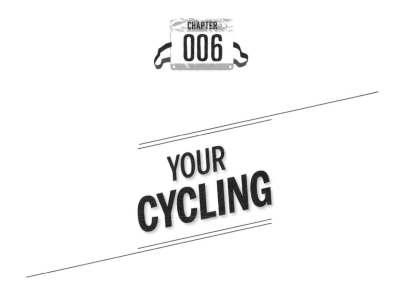

CHAPTER

006

YOUR
CYCLING

You won't cover much real estate when running and even less when swimming, but you can see a lot in an hour or so of bike riding. You'll get to know the details of the roads and the bike paths where you ride better than you ever have in your car or on foot. In a car you are insulated from the rest of the world, which goes by quickly. When walking or running, your range is pretty small. But on a bike you experience the world firsthand and travel many miles.

Many experienced triathletes consider the bike leg of a triathlon the most important because they spend about half the total race time on two wheels. In contrast with the swim and the run, the bike involves much more technology, as it's the only part of a triathlon using a machine. And since you are dealing with technology, this is also the most expensive part of getting equipped for your first triathlon.

YOUR BIKE

You don't have to ride a fancy, expensive bike to do your first triathlon. In fact, I recommend using whatever bike you already have in the garage, as long as it's safe to ride. If you're unsure about that, take it to a local bike shop and have the mechanic take a look. If you've chosen a first-timer-friendly race, you'll find lots of people riding all kinds of bikes, many of which are in disrepair. But be sure to have yours fixed up a bit. You don't want it breaking down on a long ride far from home.

Schedule your trusty steed for a tune-up. If your bike has been sitting around gathering dust, it probably needs some maintenance to make it road-ready, including chain lubrication, brake pad and tire replacement, and adjustment of all cables, bolts, and bearing races. After the tune-up you'll be surprised at how much easier—and fun!—it is to ride.

Selecting a Bike

But what if you're in the mood to buy a new bike? Again, I don't recommend doing this. Buying a bike is a tricky venture even for a seasoned triathlete. Once you have a couple of races under your belt, you'll have a much better idea of what you need in a bike. And chances are that if you do buy a new bike now, after you know more you will regret having purchased it.

Okay, I couldn't convince you, and you are determined to spend some money. So what do you buy? First decide what category of bike to purchase. There are five major categories, and each has good and bad points. You need to decide if you want a bike that will be used only for triathlons or if you also want to use it for century (100-mile) rides, tours, errands around town, or off-road riding. Tough question, huh? This is why I suggest waiting. Anyway, here are your choices and the different features of each.

TRIATHLON BIKE

If you know you're going to use the bike primarily for triathlons, which you will do several of, with maybe an occasional century or short tour, then this is the way to go. Triathlon bikes (see Figure 6.1) are made to help you go fast when riding alone. They are designed for aerodynamics and speed, not comfort. Riding one of these will put you in a low position, with your upper-body weight resting on your elbows. They may not be ridden off-road on trails at all.

> **Frame** (main triangle usually made of tubes). The upright seat tube is generally steeper (more vertical) than on other bikes to give you a slightly lower and more aerodynamic position.
>
> **Wheels.** They usually have a diameter of 700 millimeters or 27 inches. They often have a low number of spokes (16 to 32) or have a solid-looking disk wheel in the rear for aerodynamics.
>
> **Tires.** The tires are narrow and pumped to a very high pressure to give you more speed.
>
> **Gears.** Two chainrings are common in the front, although you can have a third, smaller one installed for hilly courses. Newer bikes generally have 10 gears on the rear wheel.
>
> **Handlebars.** On a tri bike the handlebars are low and narrow, and they have supports for your elbows to reduce the amount of speed-robbing drag your body creates.

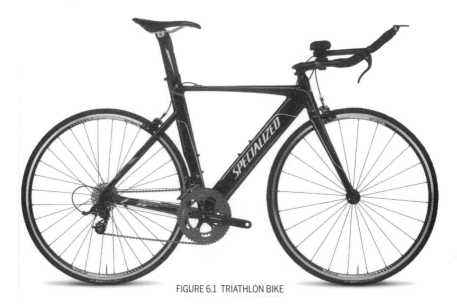

FIGURE 6.1 TRIATHLON BIKE

ROAD BIKE

The road bike (see Figure 6.2) was designed for bike racing, as in the Tour de France. It's a bit more versatile than the triathlon bike, allowing you to easily ride in tours, centuries, and even triathlons. Road bikes are more comfortable than most triathlon bikes for rides of long duration. These bikes are very responsive—like a race car—due to their short wheelbase and stiff frame design. So the first time you ride one, you may feel a little nervous about even letting go with one hand to reach for a water bottle.

Frame. The seat tube is less steep than on a tri bike. It leans backward a bit more. This helps you sit more comfortably and climb hills more powerfully.

Wheels. As on a triathlon bike, the wheels on a road bike are generally 700 millimeters or 27 inches in diameter. They usually have 32–36 spokes.

Tires. The tires are narrow and pumped to a high pressure, but they generally don't ride as hard as a tri bike's.

Gears. Just as on a tri bike, two chainrings are common in the front, but you can add a third, smaller one to make hill climbing easier. Newer bikes generally have 10 gears on the rear wheel. The gearshift levers are usually built into the brake levers.

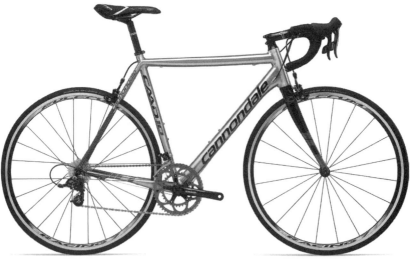

FIGURE 6.2 ROAD BIKE

Handlebars. Most road bikes come with "drop" (curved downward) handle-bars, but you can substitute straight handlebars to sit more upright and comfortably. And for a triathlon you can buy clip-on triathlon bars to lower your body and improve aerodynamics.

TOURING BIKE

The touring bike (see Figure 6.3) is much like a road bike, only with a lon-ger wheelbase and heavier design. These bikes are meant to carry packs and heavy loads. If the road bike is a race car, then the touring bike is a station wagon. It is best used in multiday century rides, but just like the road bike, it can be adapted for triathlon. This bike is comfortable but not designed for off-road use.

Frame. The seat tube angle is much like that of the road bike to improve comfort and climbing.

Wheels. With 32–36 spokes and heavier, sturdier rims, touring bike wheels are a bit more substantial than those of tri or road bikes.

Tires. The tires on touring bikes are also wider than on tri or road bikes and may have a bit more tread. The tire pressure may not be as high as that of the previous two bikes.

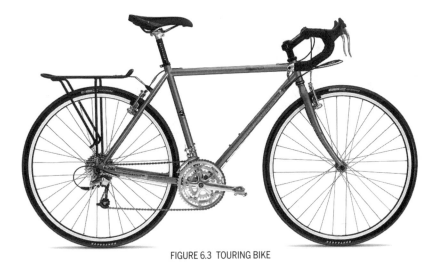

FIGURE 6.3 TOURING BIKE

Gears. Three chainrings are common, allowing you a wider range of options for going up steep hills with a heavy load or for riding comfortably on a flat section of road.

Handlebars. Most touring bikes have drop handlebars, but you can replace them with straight ones if you want to sit more upright. For a triathlon you can use clip-on bars.

MOUNTAIN BIKE

The mountain bike (see Figure 6.4) is the four-wheel-drive of bicycles. This bike is intended primarily for trail riding on rugged terrain. Most people find these bikes very comfortable because they have softer tires and often a suspension system. But mountain bikes are slow, and even slower on pavement because of their heavy, knobby tires. If you don't have to ride fast and you intend to use your bike for off-road riding as well as for running short errands, then this is a good choice. The mountain bike can be used in a triathlon just as it is. In fact, you will see a number of people riding them at your first triathlon.

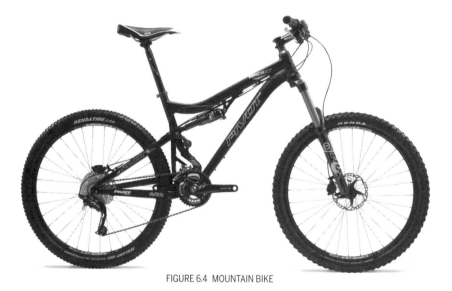

FIGURE 6.4 MOUNTAIN BIKE

Frame. These bikes are a little smaller than road or tri bikes and have a rugged design.

Wheels. In order to deal with trail riding, the wheels are even sturdier than on touring bikes and are a bit smaller, at about 26 inches or 650 millimeters in diameter. Some mountain bikes now also come with 29-inch wheels.

Tires. The tires are the widest of any of these bikes and have heavy knobs on them to improve traction on loose dirt.

Gears. With three chainrings and a wide range of gears on the rear wheel, this bike can climb very steep hills.

Handlebars. Long, straight handlebars allow you to sit upright.

HYBRID BIKE

These are the popular "fitness" bikes ridden by many people at triathlons. Hybrid bikes (see Figure 6.5) are also sometimes called "cross" bikes because they are a cross among road, touring, and mountain bikes. They can be used for errands around town, on smooth and easy trails, and in short triathlons.

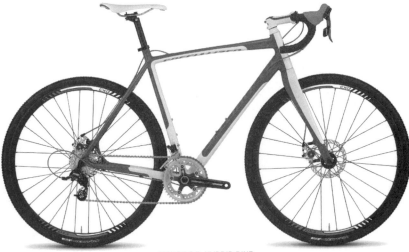

FIGURE 6.5 HYBRID BIKE

Frame. The shape is similar to a road bike's, but you sit upright as on a mountain bike. A little sturdier than a road bike, a hybrid bike isn't as heavy as a mountain bike.

Wheels. With 32–36 spokes and sturdy rims, the wheels on a hybrid bike are like those on a touring bike.

Tires. The tires are also similar to those on a touring bike.

Gears. Three chainrings are common, allowing you a wider range of options for going up steep hills with a heavy load or for riding comfortably on a flat section of road.

Handlebars. They are straight, like those on mountain bikes.

Bike Fit

No matter whether you use your old bike or buy a new one for your first triathlon, it's important that the bike fit you. Riding a bike that is too big or too small is not only uncomfortable, which means you won't look forward to training on it, but also unsafe and likely to cause injury, especially to your knees and back. So if you borrow someone else's bike, make sure it is the right size for you. To get a rough idea of proper sizing, stand over the bike with your shoes on. You should have an inch or two of clearance between your crotch and the top tube. Women typically have more difficulty with bike sizing because their torsos are short relative to their leg length when compared with men. Most bikes are made for men's sizing. A shorter handlebar stem may help to shorten the reach for a woman.

Once you have the right-size frame, you need to make sure it is set up properly for you. The best way to do this is with a bike-fit specialist— someone who actually spends time with you making adjustments. This can be a bit expensive, but if you decide to step up to a triathlon bike, I highly recommend it. For now we need to get your bike set so that it's about right. When following the bike-fit suggestions below, avoid setting the seatpost or the handlebar stem too high. There is a mark on the seatpost and the handlebars indicating their safe extension limit. Do not exceed that mark.

Before You Get in the Saddle

Believe it or not, there are right and wrong ways to sit on a bike. Many new cyclists position themselves on their bikes as if they were sitting on a bar stool and leaning on the bar. Their backs are arched like a cat's back. An arched back restricts breathing slightly, making it harder to breathe deeply while pedaling the bike fast.

To get your back in the correct position, you need to first get your pelvis right. Think of your pelvis as a bowl. In the bar stool sitting position your pelvis is level. Although that may sound comfortable (if you look past the strain on your back), it means that the big muscles of your thighs—the hamstrings and the quads—are restricted and unable to fully deliver power to the pedals. You don't want to ride a bike this way.

So how should you sit? Again, imagine your pelvis as a bowl, this time filled with water. You should sit so that the water spills out of the front side. When you sit on the bike your pelvis should be slightly tilted, with the front part of the bowl tipped lower than the rear. Sitting this way takes some practice and getting used to, but once you get it you will have a flatter back, allowing you to move more air in and out of your lungs, and your leg muscles will work more effectively.

You may find that sitting on the bike this way causes some groin discomfort. That's a sign that either your saddle isn't right for you or your bike isn't set up properly, or both. Having your bike properly set up by a fit specialist will make it easier to sit this way.

The following steps will help you get your bike set right. It's best to do this with your bike in a trainer so it is upright, level, and balanced. Ride your bike on the trainer for 10 minutes or so to get warmed up and in a comfortable position. Then start making adjustments. It's a good idea to have someone help with this.

Step 1. If you are using cleats on your bike shoes, start by positioning them so that the ball of your foot is above and slightly ahead of the pedal spindle.

Step 2. Set the saddle angle so that it is flat or parallel to the ground. Then you need to set saddle height. With your bike shoes on, place your heels on the pedals and slowly turn the cranks backward. At the bottom of the stroke your heels should still be on the pedals, with your knee locked out straight. Adjust your saddle height accordingly. Do not adjust it so high that it exceeds the maximum height mark on the seatpost.

Step 3. Adjust the saddle fore-aft position by dropping a plumb line from the front of your knee. A small weighted object on the end of a string will do this quite nicely. The plumb line should drop within a half inch in front of or behind the pedal spindle without changing your position on the saddle. If you moved the saddle either forward or backward, you will need to once again check your fore-aft position with a plumb line.

Step 4. Next, set the handlebar height so it is about 2–3 inches below the top of your saddle. Do not raise it so high that it exceeds the maximum height line engraved on the portion of the stem that goes into the head tube. Some bikes don't have a one-piece stem; instead the stem is fastened with bolts to a steering tube. This type will have spacers below the stem that are used to adjust handlebar height. For this type of stem I'd strongly recommend taking your bike to a shop for expert assistance.

Step 5. When the handlebar stem is the proper length, the handlebars should keep you from seeing the front hub as you look down from a seated position. If you are well behind or forward of this position, then either the frame is the wrong size or the stem is not the right length. In either case it's best to take the bike to a bike shop at this time for an evaluation. The staff there can change out the stem for you if necessary.

OTHER CYCLING EQUIPMENT

When you're getting ready for your first triathlon, it's important to have the right gear in all three sports, but you'll find that bicycling requires the most stuff. I like to divide triathlon bike equipment into two categories—must-have and nice-to-have.

Must-Have Equipment

This list, of course, assumes that you have a decent bike that is safe and in good working order.

HELMET

In the old days of triathlon (ca. 1985), helmets were optional. That is no longer true, and with good reason. Safety on the bike should be your paramount concern, but accidents outside of your control can, and do, happen. Race directors now require all participants to wear an approved helmet designed for use on a bicycle. This is one area in which you should not skimp on price. Choose your new helmet based first on head protection and fit and second on color and style. And then wear it whenever and wherever you ride, no matter how slow or easy you might be going. You never know when you might need it. Helmets run $50–$200.

BIKE SHORTS

You're going to spend a lot of time on your saddle as you get ready for your first triathlon. A good pair of bike shorts with a padded crotch will help the time go by quickly. Running shorts won't hack it. You need some cushioning between your rear and the saddle. Don't wear underwear beneath your bike shorts, as that defeats the purpose. Most bike shorts are black because you might have to wipe your greasy hands on them during a ride. There are two main types to choose from: loose-fitting, touring-style shorts and tight-fitting racer shorts. Either will work fine for your first triathlon, so your choice comes down to style and preference. Expect to pay $35–$200 for shorts.

PUMPS

You'll need two pumps—a frame pump for your bike and a floor pump. The frame pump is carried while you ride in case of a flat out on the road. The first time you have to use it you'll understand why I say also buy a floor pump. It's common to have to pump your tires every few days before starting a ride. Using a frame pump every time makes this a workout in itself. The floor pump just stays in your garage until needed. An alternative to a frame pump that is popular among triathletes is carrying CO_2 cartridges during a ride. These take up less space and are much easier to use when a tube needs inflating after a flat. Frame pumps cost $10–$50. CO_2 cartridges go for about $3 apiece. You'll need a device to connect the cartridge to the valve stem. These cost $15–$30 and include a cartridge to get you started. Floor pumps cost $20–$100.

GLOVES

Like bike shorts, these are another product that makes riding more comfortable. Padded gloves also protect your hands in case of a fall. And when you get really good at riding a bike, they also can be used to flick stickers and glass off your tires without stopping or cutting your hands. Fingerless gloves are best for road riding in warmer months. Gloves cost anywhere from $13 to $35.

BOTTLE CAGE

You'll want to carry water or a sports drink on your bike while training and in the race. There are several options for doing this, but the simplest and least expensive is having a bottle cage mounted on your bike. You may already have one of these, but if you don't, look to spend $7–$40.

REPAIR KIT

Chances are that someday you will get a flat tire during one of your rides. That could mean a long walk home, so carrying the basic needs for repairing a flat, and knowing how to fix it, are a necessity (see the "How to

Repair a Flat" sidebar at the end of this chapter). You can pick up a small patch kit and some tire levers in a bike shop. Also purchase a spare tube and carry it on all rides, as this is what you will go to first in case of a flat. Should you have a second flat on the same ride, you'll have to use the patch kit to repair it. It's also very helpful to have a small saddlebag that fastens under your seat to carry all this. In the saddlebag, you can carry a few dollars for an emergency phone call or a sports drink. (It's also a good idea to have a cell phone in your pocket whenever out on a ride.) Altogether, a repair kit will cost you about $30–$50.

—

You may have some equipment already, but if you were to buy all the must-haves discussed, you would spend at least $145. That may seem like a lot; however, given that you are making a long-term commitment to triathlon, you should think of it as an investment in your health, fitness, and lifestyle, not a onetime, frivolous expense.

Nice-to-Have Equipment

Now let's take a look at a few nice-to-haves. These are products that will make you faster or more comfortable or will make training easier. They are not necessities. Triathletes tend to add these items to their arsenals over time, starting soon after their first race.

BIKE JERSEY

You can ride and race in a T-shirt. A lot of people do. But a cotton T-shirt flapping in the breeze will work like a sail to slow you down, and on a hot day it holds a lot of sweat. Bike jerseys resolve those problems and provide pockets in the back to carry stuff like money, a cell phone, a spare tube or a patch kit, food, facial tissue, or anything else you want to take along. They are brightly colored to make you more visible to motorists. Jerseys run $35–$80.

HANDLEBAR COMPUTER

A no-frills handlebar computer tells you current, average, and maximum speed; distance; time; and time of day. Or you can get more bells and whistles, with heart rate, altitude, cadence, grade, night light, temperature, and more. These cost $30–$300 depending on the number of features.

MIRROR

If you plan to spend a lot of time riding your bike on public streets and roads, having a mirror helps you ride more safely and provides some peace of mind about what is coming up behind you. With a mirror you can keep your eye on traffic without turning your head, which can be tricky at times, and you can also see others riding behind you. Mirrors fasten either to your helmet or to the end of your handlebars. They cost $5–$20.

BIKE SHOES

This one could really be in either category. Once you have your first triathlon behind you, put this on your must-have list. For now you can ride in running shoes, and lots of new triathletes do. But because they are flexible and soft, running shoes not only make you lose power but also can cause your feet to get sore on longer rides. When you are training for your first sprint or Olympic triathlon your rides won't be all that long.

You have two choices in shoes—road and touring. Road shoes are stiffer, allowing you to transfer more power to the pedals (see the description of clipless pedals) on each stroke. It's a good idea to purchase your road shoes and clipless pedals together. The drawback is that road shoes are hard to walk around in, though that's generally not a problem for triathletes. But if you also want to use the same shoes when doing centuries and tours, then touring shoes may be better since they are a bit more flexible and easier to walk in. Shoes cost about $60–$300.

CLIPLESS PEDALS

Your bike may have come with toe clips, an adjustable strap that goes around your foot to hold it in place. These work fine, but clipless pedals can be much easier to get in and out of once you get used to them. Much like ski bindings, you just twist your foot and it pops out. This setup allows you to quickly get your foot back in the pedal, and being clipped in gives you more power and efficiency. Do make sure you allow yourself plenty of time to get comfortable with your clipless pedals before you ride in traffic. Expect to pay $50–$330.

INDOOR TRAINER

If you live someplace that is really cold in the winter or really hot in the summer, you may want to consider buying an indoor trainer. This is a small device that you mount your bike on. It provides resistance against the rear wheel so that the effort is very much like being out on the open road. It uses a small fan, a magnet, or encased fluid to create the resistance. Trainers allow you to get a ride in when the weather, traffic, darkness, kids, or even a good show on TV wouldn't otherwise allow it. Trainers cost $130–$550.

AEROBARS

If you want to race faster in a triathlon, this is the ticket. Aerobars put you into a low, aerodynamic position with your elbows resting on pads and your hands outstretched in front. You can buy either one-piece aerobars or clip-ons that you simply clamp on to your existing handlebars. It's best to have someone experienced with bike setup do this for you. That could be a mechanic at the shop where you buy the bars. Aerobars cost $50–$700.

SPECIAL WHEELS

Next to having aerobars, special wheels will do the most to make you go fast. You can find some that are solid, called "disk wheels," but I don't recommend those for your first triathlon. In fact, most triathletes should put off this purchase for several seasons. Look for those that have 32 or fewer spokes to a wheel. The fewer spokes, the less "eggbeater" effect on the air as you travel through it. This means faster speed due to reduced drag. "Fast" wheels can be a big expense, but they are more than likely something you will eventually want. Look to spend at least $200–$300 for a pair of good wheels.

BASIC CYCLING SKILLS

You've probably been riding a bike for a long time, but you might find that the basic cycling skills take on new meaning as you begin riding farther and faster. Here's a quick primer in the skills and techniques involved.

Braking and Stopping

First things first. The rear brake is operated with the right hand and the front brake with the left hand. The front brake has more stopping power than the rear, but used alone in an emergency situation it may cause you to flip over the handlebars. The rear brake is best for slowing you down gradually and should always be used in conjunction with the front brake. Apply the rear brake to gradually slow the bike, and then the front brake when it's time to stop.

Shifting Gears

You'll hear the phrases "high gear" and "low gear" a lot in cycling. A high gear is one that slows down your cadence (revolutions per minute) and causes you to rely more heavily on muscle to turn the cranks. A low gear does just the opposite—it increases your cadence, making you breathe harder. When riding you always want to find the best gear for the current conditions—hills, wind, and how fresh you are feeling. Simply shifting to a higher or a lower gear sometimes makes the effort feel easier.

There are two sets of gears on your bike. Those in the front, close to the pedals, are called chainrings. The gears on the rear wheel are called cogs. The highest gears use the big chainring, while the lowest gears use the small chainring. The cogs on the rear wheel work in just the opposite way. The bigger the gear, the easier it is to turn the pedals, and the smaller the gear, the harder it is to turn them. So by combining big or small chainrings with bigger or smaller cogs on the rear wheel, you can create many different combinations to fine-tune the effort you put out while pedaling.

There are a couple of combinations you won't want to use, however. It's best not to use the big chainring with the largest cog on the back wheel, the one closest to the spokes. Nor should you combine the small chainring with the smallest cog on the rear wheel, the one farthest from the spokes. These gearing combinations are called "crossover," meaning that the chain is running at an extreme angle from front to back. This increases the wear and tear on the chain and the gears, causing them to need replacing sooner.

Cornering and Turning

One of the most dangerous maneuvers on a ride, especially a fast one, is negotiating corners.

The first rule of cornering is, don't brake in the corner. If the turn is free of gravel and water you should be able to take it at full speed by leaning. But if it's necessary to slow down, brake before you get into the turn. Then let go of the brake levers as the turn begins.

The most important moment in taking a corner safely is the early part. If the speed and the line you selected are right, you will have no problems. Practice approaching corners at various speeds. Make it second nature to judge how fast to take them. The line you select depends on speed. A fast speed requires a more gradual and sweeping turn than does slow cornering.

Sit in the middle of your saddle, not on the nose or back end of it. This will help you maintain balance. As the turn starts, stop pedaling so that your inside knee is high, put most of your weight on the outside pedal, and lean to the inside. The faster you are going, the more you should lean. The lean of the bike should be greater than the lean of your upper body. To accomplish this, keep your head upright so that the line of your eyes is parallel to the road surface. Don't lean your head into the turn. When the bike becomes more upright as you exit the corner, begin to pedal again.

Hone your cornering skills by going to a parking lot or other area with no traffic and practicing left and right turns until you become comfortable with both. Right turns are simple. Signal your intention before arriving at the corner. Check for pedestrians who might step out in front of you. Then stay to the right but away from the very edge of the road as you make the turn. Left turns are a lot trickier. If the street you are on has a dedicated left-turn lane, check traffic approaching from behind, signal you are going left, and then move to the right side of the left-turn lane. Cross when traffic clears and the light is green. For a multilane street with no dedicated left-turn lane, stop on the right side and wait for a break in traffic before crossing. Or make a 90-degree turn by riding straight across the intersection to the far corner. Stop to check traffic on the street you were on and then cross the intersection so you are proceeding in the desired direction.

Climbing and Descending

There's no doubt that riding up hills will make you a stronger bike rider. While riding on a flat stretch of road, you can ease up anytime. But when climbing a hill, letting up may cause you to fall over. You have to reach down deep to find the power to keep going on steep hills. Although they are hard and perhaps even frustrating at first, hills will soon become your strongest ally in the quest to become a better rider.

On hills the trick is to find the right gear combination. New riders tend to select a high gear, stand, and "muscle" the bike up the hill. This puts a lot of stress on the knees and can result in injury. Try to find a gearing combination that allows you to stay seated and spin with a bit higher cadence. It may help to have your bike shop put a third chainring on your bicycle if you find that getting over hills is extremely difficult. Compact chainrings are another option to give you lower gears without the extra chainring. As you approach a hill, allow your momentum to carry you up a few yards. Then shift quickly to a lower gear. Using the right one for you on any given hill will soon become second nature. But at first you'll need to experiment a bit.

Your position on the bike when going up a hill is a bit different than when riding on flat roads. If you have triathlon aerobars or road drop/hooked bars, place your hands on the top portion of the handlebars near the stem. Although this will make you less aerodynamic, it will give you more power. Wind resistance is less important than power on a hill. It may also help to scoot your rear a little farther back on the saddle so you can push a bit forward with the pedals rather than straight down. Again, this makes you more powerful.

Descending a steep hill can be scary even for the most experienced bike riders. As your bike-handling skills get better you'll find that your speed on descents increases. But at first it's okay to gently "feather" the rear brake when it feels as if you're starting to go too fast. There is no fitness to be gained from coming down a hill, but there is a lot to be lost. So sit up to create wind break, hold a straight line, concentrate on where you want to go, keep your hands on the brake levers, feather the brakes a bit, and be conservative.

Pedaling

The skill of pedaling a bike seems fairly simple. After all, your feet are on the pedals, which are attached to the crank arms revolving around a fixed point at the bottom bracket. What could go wrong? Actually, quite a bit. Sports scientists have shown that there are differences in pedaling ability among even experienced athletes. These differences mean that some riders are more efficient than others. Those who pedal most smoothly gain their efficiency primarily at the top and the bottom of the pedal circle. Learning to pedal more like them means that you can go faster with the same effort or that you can ride easier at the same speed.

Anyone can push down on the pedal correctly because the way we are built and gravity combine to make the pedal go from top to bottom easily.

The tricky parts are the top and the bottom of the stroke. These are a bit more difficult to get right, but if you do, riding will be a whole lot more fun. So let's figure out the top and bottom parts of the pedal stroke.

The reason the top and the bottom are so tricky has to do with changes in direction. As your foot and pedal are approaching the top of the stroke, your leg has to change direction, from going back and up to going forward and down. As your foot and pedal approach the bottom of the stroke, the opposite has to happen. These changes, or "transitions," are difficult to get right, especially the top one. Do them wrong and you waste energy—something you can't afford to do when riding hard in a triathlon.

So how do you make the transitions smooth? Watch your foot position on the pedal and train your muscles. When pedaling, your heel should be slightly (about half an inch) higher than the ball of your foot. This angles your foot just enough so that the transitions are easier. To train your muscles to work correctly, work these drills into the first few minutes of every ride. When you are warming up, your legs will be fresh and you can focus better on technique. These drills concentrate mostly on the top transition, because it is the more difficult one.

ISOLATED LEG-TRAINING DRILL

This is best done on an indoor trainer because it's a bit risky on the road. Unclip one foot from the pedal and place it on a chair or a box next to the bike. Then, with the bike in a low and easy gear, pedal with the other leg. You'll find that at the top of the pedal stroke there is a "dead" spot that is a bit difficult to pedal through. Focus on this dead spot to smooth it out. Change legs when the working leg fatigues—you might last only a few seconds. Over time you will become more efficient at the top of the stroke and be able to pedal longer before tiring. This is a sign that your pedal transitions are improving.

9-TO-3 DRILL

This and all the following drills are done with both feet clipped into the pedals and may be used on the road or indoor trainer. In the 9-to-3 drill, think of the pedal stroke as being the face of a clock, with 12 o'clock at the top and 6 o'clock at the bottom. When the crank arms are parallel to the ground, the forward foot is in the 3 o'clock position and the back foot is at 9 o'clock. You want to feel as if you are moving your rear foot straight forward from 9 to 3 on the clock face without ever going through 12. Obviously you are, but by firing the muscles this way you train them to transition smoothly. Every minute or so, think about pedaling this way for several seconds. Take a mental break and then do it again. This is especially helpful early in your warm-up, but you can repeat it throughout the ride to check on your pedaling technique.

SHOE-TOP DRILL

This one is a bit challenging, but great for getting the transitions right. As you are pedaling, try to keep the top of your foot pressed against the inside of your shoe. Avoid touching the bottom inside of your shoe. This drill emphasizes all parts of the pedal stroke except the downstroke, which is the easy part.

TOE-TOUCH DRILL

The toe-touch drill concentrates on the top transition. As your foot approaches the 12 o'clock position, try to touch your toes to the front end of your shoe. Make sure your heel is slightly higher than the ball of your foot when doing this.

SPIN-UP DRILL

Cadence, how many pedal strokes one foot completes in a minute, has a lot to do with how efficiently you pedal. Each of us has a comfortable cadence range. When your cadence falls below your comfortable range, you feel as if you are using too much muscle to push down. When it is higher than your comfortable range, you begin breathing too hard for how fast you are going. Efficient riders tend to have higher ranges than do inefficient riders. The spin-up drill is easy. Gradually increase your cadence for about 20–30 seconds until you start to bounce on the saddle. Then reduce your cadence slightly until you stop bouncing, and pedal as smoothly as you can for a few seconds at a high cadence. Repeat this drill several times during the warm-up. With practice you will become more comfortable riding at higher cadences, which improves your efficiency.

BIKE SAFETY

This is the part where I say "don't" a lot. I'll start now: Don't take safety for granted. You want to have fun and to become a better person because of triathlon. A crash can stop that in a heartbeat. Safety, safety, safety!

Riding a bike on the open road with traffic is scary—and with good reason. It's a bit like being a mouse in an elephant stampede. Almost every week I hear of a cyclist who has a bad accident, the worst of which are bike-car accidents. The most common reason for these is inattentiveness of either the bike rider or the driver—or both. You have no control over drivers, but when in or near traffic *you* must always be attentive. Don't assume the drivers are. In fact, assume they aren't and that they don't even see you. Chances are you will be right.

Never take needless risks on the road. It is better to stop fully (with a foot on the ground) while watching to see what drivers are going to do at an intersection than to bolt through it to keep your workout going. Always ride with your eyes looking ahead and scanning the area around you, not down at your front wheel because of fatigue or a determination to ride faster. You need to know what's just up the road and what drivers and other riders are doing. Don't become a statistic for the sake of fitness. All it takes is a second of inattentiveness.

Although bike-car accidents are usually the most devastating, they are not the most common. Falls account for perhaps half of all bike accidents. The next big category is bicycle-bicycle collisions. Dogs, obstacles, and other causes make up the remainder. Most of these are under your control: choose your course wisely, ride defensively, have good skills, make sure your bike is road-ready, and be attentive to what's going on around you.

Maintaining Your Equipment

Always wear a helmet. Enough said.

A common cause of accidents is not having the wheels securely fastened to the bike. A wheel wobbling in the frame and coming loose on a descent could be catastrophic. If your wheels lock on with bolts, make sure the nuts are tight. If you have quick-release skewers, it should take quite a bit of effort to close the lever all the way.

Be sure that your tires are fully inflated before every ride. Check the tread to ensure there isn't a small piece of glass or wire stuck in it. Look to see if the thread is showing on your tires. If it is, replace them immediately. If your tires are old from sitting in the garage for a long time, they may be cracked and should be replaced. There should be no bulges in the sidewall.

Check your brakes frequently. The levers should not touch the handlebars. If they do, have a mechanic adjust them. The brake pads should touch the metal wheel rims, not the tires. If they touch the tires even a little bit, the tire will blow out. Replace the brake pads when the vertical wear lines are worn off.

Lean heavily on your handlebar ends before starting a ride to make sure they don't slip. They should be very securely fastened to the stem. There should be plugs on the ends of your bars.

Visibility

Since you want to be seen by drivers, wear bright clothing. Neutral or muted colors are not generally the best choice. It helps to have a mirror either on your helmet or on the handlebars. However, you will still have blind spots and will need to check them before changing lanes or turning. Riding at dusk or dawn is not recommended, but a lot of triathletes do this, especially in the winter when daylight is limited, in order to get in their training miles. Bright headlights, taillights, and reflectors are necessities at these times. Riding indoors on a trainer is much safer.

Where to Ride

Always remember that riding a bike is a lot different than driving a car. This is most evident when you're deciding where to ride. It's best to avoid riding on busy streets, at rush hour, in the dark, on streets that have no bike lanes, and against traffic on one-way streets. The safest places to ride are usually bike paths and wide roads with little traffic. As you drive around in your car, make a mental note of the best places to ride. Then plan your routes accordingly. At certain times of the day it may be best not to ride outside at all due to traffic, darkness, or foul weather. This is when having an indoor trainer (see "Other Cycling Equipment" in this chapter) comes in very handy.

Scout two types of safe bike courses you can ride. Some of the courses should be fairly flat—as flat as you can find where you live. These will be used on days when you want to keep it easy, to develop a good base of aerobic fitness, or to work on race-type riding. Also have a hilly course or two, with grades that challenge you a bit just to get over them. Later in your training we will use these to make you stronger.

Riding in Traffic

Always ride to the side of the road in the same direction traffic is flowing. Don't ride on the sidewalk. Stay about 12–18 inches left of the edge of the road. This may seem counterintuitive, but hugging the edge encourages drivers, especially on narrow roads, to squeeze between you and oncoming traffic. If you stay a few inches to the left of the edge, they are more likely to wait for a safer moment to pass, and you have room to maneuver.

Whether you are riding in traffic or with a group, always try to ride in a predictable manner. This generally means holding a straight line so that motorists (or other cyclists) are relatively sure of your intent. Keep at least one hand on the handlebars at all times. Learn where your water bottle on the frame is located so you don't have to take your eyes off the road to grab it. The same goes for putting it back in the cage; a quick glance is all it should take.

STOP SIGNS AND STOPLIGHTS

Don't assume you have the right-of-way even if the light is green. Make sure all cars that could intersect your path are stopped before crossing the street. Be patient. Stop-and-go lights that are controlled by sensors often don't "see" bicycles. You must either wait for a car to trip the sensor or get off your bike and press the pedestrian crosswalk button.

LEFT-HAND TURNS AND LANE CHANGES

Perhaps the trickiest move for any cyclist, including a very experienced cyclist, is looking over the left shoulder to check traffic when turning or changing lanes. The bike will start drifting left if you aren't careful to counter that motion. To avoid this, lock your left elbow and slightly bend your right elbow. This position will keep your bike on a straight course.

Hand Signals

It's always a good idea to alert others that you are turning by using hand signals. This helps drivers and others riding with you know what to expect. Commonly accepted hand signals follow:

- **Stopping.** Left arm extended down with hand open and palm facing backward. In some places raising a hand overhead when riding in a group indicates stopping.
- **Left turn.** Left arm extended and pointing left.
- **Right turn.** This one varies a bit from state to state. For drivers in all states and cyclists in most, the left elbow is bent with the hand pointing straight up. In other states cyclists can simply point right with an extended right arm.

Although a mirror can help eliminate a lot of this turning, you'll still need to turn your head for a final check before moving left.

OBSTACLES

You are bound to encounter obstacles in the bike lane or on the bike path. These can cause falls and flat tires. If you're unsure about whether you can negotiate a large obstruction, it's best to stop, get off your bike, and walk around it. For smaller ones you can make slight changes in your course to avoid them. If you're riding with a group, be sure to point at any obstacles on the course to warn trailing riders.

Parked cars present a unique problem when you are riding on the right side. Check to see which cars have people in them who may open the door at the last second. Give these cars a wide berth after checking traffic over your left shoulder. If you're unsure, give a car a bit of extra space regardless. Don't weave in and out of parked cars, as drivers behind you may not see you or may misunderstand your intent.

When approaching railroad tracks that intersect the street at greater or less than a 90-degree angle, alter your course so that you cross the tracks at close to a right angle to prevent getting your front wheel twisted. Also, as you cross railroad tracks or very rough sections of road, stand on your pedals with your knees and elbows slightly bent. This will reduce the shock to your body and the bike and also will help prevent pinch flats.

DOGS

Dogs who chase will usually leave you alone as soon as you are past their "territory." It's best to pedal fast in a straight line, with both hands on the handlebars, rather than to try to hit the dog with a frame pump or squirt it with a water bottle. You might also try shouting, "Sit!" since the dog may be trained to obey that command.

Group Rides

Riding on the roads with a group makes it even more fun to be out on your bike. But before going out with a group know how fast they ride and what their purpose is. Some groups are for racers, and they ride fast and aggressively. It's best to avoid this type. Others are more social; they ride more slowly with possibly even coffee or breakfast stops. There may even be triathletes who ride together, including those who are new to the sport and want to learn more. Your bike shop can tell you more about the groups in your area and suggest the best one for you.

Riding in a group, although fun, can be dangerous. Large groups that dominate the roadway and disobey stop signs tend to make drivers angry and impatient. That's not a good combination. You also need to be more attentive to what's going on around you—such as traffic and obstacles—because you can't see as much. On the other hand, a well-led and disciplined group can make riding safer than when you're alone since you are easier for drivers to see.

You can also learn a lot from riding with experienced cyclists, including tips for training and racing and bike handling, and updates on the local triathlon scene. This is your chance to meet others with common interests and to become a better rider.

How to Repair a Flat

When you're riding along and suddenly your bike seems to be handling differently, there's a good chance that your tire is going flat. Slow leaks, rather than sudden blowouts, are the most common type of flat. Try to stop riding before the tire is completely out of air or you will be riding on the rim, causing further damage to your bike. Blowouts where the tire suddenly goes completely flat are scarier and frequently occur because of a worn tire. For this reason you should check the wear on your tires weekly. If you can see the threads of the tire, it's time to replace it.

Here are the steps for getting your tire ready to go again. It's a good idea to practice fixing a flat a few times in your garage before you are forced to do it 10 miles from home. Of course you can always carry a cell phone and call

CONTINUED

CONTINUED

someone to pick you up. This is highly recommended. Then you can repair the flat in the comfort of your garage. But here's how to fix the flat wherever you may be.

1. **Remove the wheel from the bike.** This is when having quick releases rather than bolts with nuts comes in handy. You will probably have to open the brake calipers at the wheel by pulling up on the small handle on the side. If it's the front wheel, you may need to unscrew the quick release quite a few turns, since newer bikes often have safety tabs to prevent the wheel from coming out accidentally. If it's the rear wheel, shift gears so that you are in the smallest cog on the wheel. This will make it easier to reinstall the wheel.

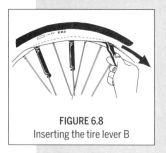

FIGURE 6.6
Deflating the tire

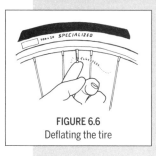

FIGURE 6.7
Inserting the tire lever A

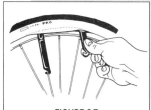

FIGURE 6.8
Inserting the tire lever B

2. **Remove only one side of the tire from the rim.** Start by making sure all the air is out of the tire by opening and pressing the inner tube valve (Figure 6.6). Then insert a tire lever under one side of the tire on the opposite side from the valve and pry the tire off (Figures 6.7 and 6.8). Slide the tire lever either forward or backward along the rim to remove more of the tire from the rim. If you can't slide the lever, pry a second part of the tire loose two or three inches from the original spot by using the other lever. This will loosen a wider part of the tire, and you should be able to slide a lever and remove one side of the tire all the way around the wheel.

3. **Remove the tube.** If there is a nut on the valve stem, take it off. Reach inside the tire and pull out the tube, removing it entirely from the wheel and tire (Figure 6.9). Maintain the tube's original orientation with the wheel in case you have to figure out where the puncture is.

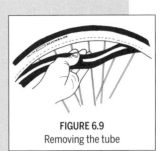

FIGURE 6.9
Removing the tube

4. **Find the puncture.** There are two types of punctures. One is caused by a sharp object such as a piece of glass or thorn penetrating the tire and tube. By slowly running your fingers around the inside of the tire while examining the outside at the same time you can often find and remove this sharp object. The other type is called a "pinch flat" and commonly occurs when the tire is underinflated. If there isn't enough air pressure, when you hit an obstacle such as railroad tracks or a pothole the tube is pinched against both sides of the rim, causing two small holes that look like a snakebite. If you don't find a sharp object, chances are you have a pinch flat, which you can confirm by finding the holes. If they aren't immediately obvious, pump some air into the tube and slowly pass it by your ear, listening for escaping air. If you find two holes there, it was a pinch. If there is only one, it was a sharp object puncture. If you kept the tube's orientation with the tire, you should now be able to examine the area where the puncture occurred to make sure there is no glass, thorn, or other sharp object that may puncture the spare tube when it's installed.

If you don't have a spare tube, your only option is to patch the puncture. Using the sandpaper in your patch kit, roughen the area around the puncture to a size a little larger than a quarter. Then apply a thin coat of rubber cement from the patch kit to an area slightly larger than the

CONTINUED

CONTINUED

patch. Allow the cement to dry for several minutes. It is dry when it no longer glistens. Without touching the contact area, remove the patch from the foil and carefully lay it on the cemented area. Use your thumbs and fingers to press the patch into place, working from the center of the patch toward the edges to release air pockets. Once it is patched, put a little bit of air into the tube to make sure it holds and check the tube for other punctures. You can also get patches that don't require cement. Check around at bike shops for these, as they will make fixing a flat out on the road much easier.

5. **Install the spare or repaired tube.** Put just enough air in the spare tube to give it a limp shape. If you are using CO_2 cartridges, rather than risk emptying the cartridge, use your mouth to blow a little air into the tube. Remove the nut, if there is one, from the valve stem. Insert the valve stem into the rim hole first. Then fit the tube into the open side of the tire all the way around.

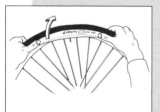

FIGURE 6.10
Putting the tire back on the rim A

6. **Put the tire back into place on the rim.** Start by pushing the valve stem up into the tire casing and allowing it to settle into position on its own (Figure 6.10). Then, starting at the valve stem and using your thumbs, push the tire back into the rim, working away from the valve stem in both directions at the same time. When you get to the last few inches of tire, deflate the tube entirely. This will make it easier to finish it off. Reinstalling the last few inches is the hardest part of the entire project. It's best to do this using only the heels of your hands by rolling the

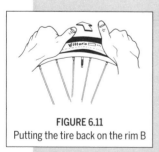

FIGURE 6.11
Putting the tire back on the rim B

tire bead up and toward the rim (Figure 6.11). If you can't get it to pop into place, carefully use a tire lever to do so, being sure not to pinch the tube against the rim.

7. **Pump up the tube.** Put just enough air in the tube to give it shape and then examine the tire all the way around to make sure no tube is protruding from under the tire. This will cause another flat. Once you are certain the tube is properly installed, pump it to the pressure rating on the side of the tire. If you're using a hand pump you'll have to guess this based on feel. And more than likely you'll fatigue long before getting there. That's all right. Just make sure that you have enough pressure in it that you don't get a pinch flat. If you're using a CO_2 cartridge, put all the gas into the tube by holding the cartridge handle fully depressed until there is no more gas coming out. CO_2 cartridges make inflating a tire a breeze.

8. **Replace the wheel on the bike.** If it's the front wheel, slip it into place, making sure it is centered between the brake pads, and then screw the quick release or the nut back into place. If it's the rear wheel, pull the rear derailleur backward and place the chain on the smallest cog. Let go of the derailleur and slip the wheel into the dropout slots. Center the wheel between the brake pads and tighten the quick release lever. In either case, be sure to push the lever on the brake caliper down to properly space the brakes from the rim.

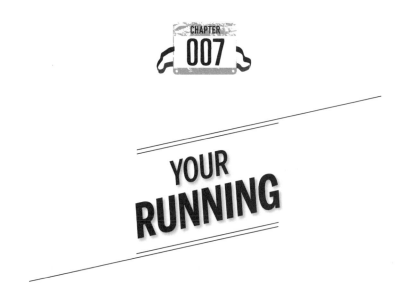

CHAPTER

007

YOUR
RUNNING

The third leg of your first triathlon—the run—is often the most challenging for new triathletes. To fully develop the fitness necessary to run three or six miles nonstop may take several months rather than just a few weeks, as we are planning to do here. So if you are completely new to running, your goal for this segment of the triathlon will be to finish it vertically with a smile on your face. I don't care how long it takes or how much you may walk. No worries, mate!

If you are an experienced runner, your run mileage will drop as you integrate swimming and biking into your weekly routine. Don't let that bother you. You'll keep the harder run days and use the swim and the bike as "recovery" workouts. You may well run faster (and avoid injury) as a result.

GOOD RUNNING FORM

Believe it or not, most people do not know how to run. In some cases they have even been instructed to run incorrectly by "experts." The quickest way to learn to run using proper form is to run barefoot on grass. Go to a park, pick out a flat or slightly downhill stretch of grass that is about 100 yards long, and inspect it to make sure it is free of debris such as broken glass, animal droppings, and thorns. Then take off your shoes and run quickly over your grassy course. Turn and walk back to where you began. Repeat this three to five more times. This workout is called "strides." (See Run Workouts 8 and 20 in Appendix A.)

What you will find when running shoeless is that your running changes in two small, but very significant, ways. The first noticeable change is that you don't land on your heels; you land with the foot more or less "flat" on the ground with the weight toward the ball of your foot. Also, because you are landing on a flat foot instead of on your heel, you will most likely take more steps to cover the distance than with shoes on—and you'll be faster as a result.

So why does your form change so much when you take off your shoes? The design of running shoes, with an elevated, padded heel, encourages you to land on the back end of your foot. It just seems logical with so much rubber there. Even when you are consciously trying to land correctly, the elevated heel makes it difficult to place your foot flat. When you land on your heel it means you must roll forward over the entire length of your foot—from the heel to the ball—before pushing off the big toe for the next stride. Research shows that the longer the foot is in contact with the ground, the slower you run. Fast runners spend very little time on the ground compared with runners at the back of the pack. They put their feet down flat and immediately spring off them. In fact, when you land with a flat foot and your weight toward the forefoot, a natural recoil effect is created in your calf muscle. This quickly captures and releases the "potential" energy, springing you up and forward and thus saving some "biological" energy, mostly carbohydrates, a scarce energy source.

You can experience this by standing with your knees bent and feet side by side and then hopping up and down on the balls of your feet.

It's an almost effortless motion. Now try doing the same thing on your heels. Notice how much more energy it takes to hop. What you experience on the balls of your feet is the elastic energy of your calf muscles. A flat footstrike makes running easier and more efficient because you are staying off your heels.

The trick is to figure out how to transfer your natural barefoot running form to fully shod running, which is certainly what you will do in your first triathlon. This takes some dedicated practice. Every time you go for a run-walk workout (with shoes on), use the feel of the barefoot technique you experienced on grass. Put your foot down flat on the ground. Do not try to land on your toes or the balls of your feet. This will almost always lead to injury for new runners. This flat footstrike will take concentration initially, but the first several runs in the training plan are quite short to allow you to focus on the technique.

If you have been running for a long time, it will be more difficult to improve your technique. There are more strides workouts on grass in the plan for experienced runners. At first these should be the only run workouts in which you use the barefoot technique. But after four of these you should be ready to use the proper form in the first 10 minutes of each run before returning to your old form. Over time increase the duration of the flat footstrike technique. Adjust your running intervals at the first sign of calf, Achilles, or foot problems. It may take longer for you to change your form than it does for the complete beginner, but give it a try. I think you will find that the flat-footed landing ultimately makes running easier.

BUILDING FITNESS FOR NEW RUNNERS

For the triathlete who is new to running, there is a lot of walking scheduled in the training plans found in Chapter 9. This will help prevent the soreness that almost always comes with starting to run for the first time. Combining walking with running is a lot easier on your body, and yet it will still produce the necessary fitness gains.

The running schedule I created also calls for interval training right from the start. Running authorities usually frown on this for novices, but in my experience newbies make greater gains when the exercise session is broken into alternating walk and run periods. At first the run portions will be short, with long walk breaks, but soon the walking gets shorter as the run duration is extended. The key here is for you to pay attention to how your legs feel. If soreness persists for more than 48 hours after running, you weren't ready for it. Return to only walking in this situation.

STAYING HEALTHY

If you get injured while training for your first triathlon, running will most likely be the culprit. The reason for this is the stress placed on your legs by pounding the pavement. Also, when running, your leg muscles are used differently than in the other two sports. The big muscles of the legs—for example, the thigh and the calf—lengthen at the same time they are trying to shorten during the running stride. They are literally being pulled apart. Sports scientists call this "eccentric contraction." Because of the pounding and eccentric contractions, runners have a higher likelihood of injury than bike riders and swimmers do.

Common Causes of Injuries

For a triathlete, nothing is worse than an injury. Not only is there discomfort, but there is also a feeling of frustration as hard-earned fitness erodes while you sit around waiting for the injury to heal. Those new to running are prone to experience sore knees, shin and foot discomfort, and other minor aches and pains. Among the worst injuries for runners are stress fractures (foot and shin), patellar tendinitis (knee), patellofemoral syndrome (knee), plantar fasciitis (foot), and iliotibial band syndrome (knee). If you develop one of these injuries, your medical provider will probably suggest you stop running until it heals. That could be several weeks if you didn't catch it soon enough.

There are typically four causes of running injuries. The first is poor technique, addressed previously in this chapter. But your technique may also be related to a second cause—weakness or inflexibility. It takes at least several months for the muscles of the legs and feet to adapt to the proper technique. During this adjustment period all the leg and foot muscles, both the large and the small ones, along with the tendons and bones, are going through changes. There are also adaptations taking place in the upper body from the hips through the entire back. You can't rush these changes. They just take time. The training schedules described in Chapter 9 address this issue by starting you into running gradually. Don't try to make the fitness happen faster. Be patient.

A third cause of injury is running in improper shoes. Later in this chapter I'll tell you how to go about finding the right shoes, but for now the message is this: Don't run in basketball, aerobics, gym, or any other type of shoe not designed for running. Get the proper equipment for the sport. You'll progress faster and have a much lower risk of injury.

A fourth common cause of running injuries is inherited traits such as flat feet or leg-length differences. Flat feet are quite common and are likely to require a special type of shoe or even orthotics (specially made insoles that can help correct imbalances). How do you know if you have flat feet? Look at your wet footprint on the tile floor after you step out of the shower. If you can see that your arch touched the floor, leaving a "bear paw" impression, then you have flat feet. Other, less common foot problems may also promote injury. It's best to see a sports medicine doctor or podiatrist if you suspect you may be dealing with any of these issues.

The same is true for leg-length differences. If you keep getting injured in one leg, your legs may be significantly different in length. This sets you up for a unique set of stresses. It's best to see a medical professional, such as a physical therapist, if this is the case.

Running on hard surfaces may complicate any of these causes. Excessive training, especially when combined with inadequate rest, is often the "final straw" that results in injury. That's why the suggested training plans in Chapter 9 have you start off so easy with running—I don't want you to get injured.

Injury Prevention

Proper technique, softer running surfaces, good equipment, gradual training increases, stretching, and muscular strength are the best safeguards against injury. Adequate recovery time following workouts, as prescribed in Chapter 9, is also necessary to stay injury-free.

If all this fails, take immediate action. At the first sign of soreness during a workout, stop and walk home. Don't push through unusual discomfort thinking it will go away by itself. Pain is your body's way of telling you "too much."

Should a suspected injury occur, here are the steps to take:

1. *Rest the injured area.* Stay off it as much as you can. Don't try to stretch it for at least the first 24 hours, or to test its condition with even limited activity.

2. *Apply ice immediately.* This can be done with an ice pack (bags of frozen corn or peas make great ice packs) or water frozen in a foam cup (if using the cup, massage the area gently). In either case, apply the ice for about 15 minutes at a time. If using an ice bag, place a thin washcloth over the skin to prevent frostbite.

3. *Compress it.* With some types of injury, such as a sprained ankle, wrapping an elastic bandage around the area snugly will help control swelling. Be careful not to cut off circulation. If there is noticeable swelling, see your doctor immediately.

4. *Elevate it.* Keep the injured area above your heart as much as possible. This helps control swelling.

If the injury doesn't respond to such treatment in the first five days even though you've stopped running, it's time to see your doctor. For some injuries you may be referred to a specialist, such as a podiatrist, orthopedist, or physical therapist.

Group Running

Should you run with a group or by yourself? There are advantages and disadvantages either way. If you have a hard time getting motivated for a run, then a small group is for you. Knowing friends are waiting for you is generally all it takes to get those running shoes on. Be careful of joining groups that like to make training runs into mini-races. These groups will push you to go too fast and might soon cause you to break down in some way with sore muscles, injury, or fatigue. For now your run workouts should be quite easy. Look for others who share that point of view.

The best groups are generally those organized weekly by running clubs, running stores, or health clubs. These will often break up the crowd into smaller groups by ability, scout out a safe course, and may even provide sports drinks along the way. Ask around to find a group that is right for you. You may need to make some changes to the suggested training plan in Chapter 9 to fit into the group. That's okay.

WHERE TO RUN

One of the best ways to avoid injuries is to run on softer surfaces such as gravel roads, dirt shoulders of paved roads, running tracks, dirt trails, and grass. These surfaces will absorb some of the impact so it doesn't wreak havoc with your legs and feet. If you prefer pavement, select asphalt over concrete. Both are hard surfaces, but asphalt is a bit softer than concrete.

Also be careful running on terrain that is always sloping in the same direction, either to your left or to your right. This is common when running in the street facing traffic, with the gutter on your left. Sidewalks also generally have a slight cant sloping downward toward the street. Canted surfaces will put uneven stress on your legs. If side-sloping running routes are unavoidable, at least try to mix them up so you get cants in both directions during a single run. That said, it's best not to have your back to traffic if you are running in the street.

As your running fitness improves, some of the workouts in Chapter 9 will include hills. Running uphill is one of the most effective ways to improve fitness because it forces you to work hard. You use more muscle, your heart rate increases, and your breathing becomes faster and more labored. But be careful on the downhill portions of your run, especially if you are on pavement. The pounding of normal running will be greatly magnified but the fitness gains will be minimal. So go slowly on downhills. It's okay to walk.

If possible you should have two types of running courses—a flat one and a hilly one. But what if you live on the coast of Florida or someplace similar where there are no hills, or you live in Colorado's Rocky Mountains, where there are no long stretches of flat terrain? One of the best options is treadmill running. Treadmills are also a great alternative when the weather is too nasty to go outside. These running machines not only allow you to have convenient hills and flats but also give you control over pace, with feedback on how fast you are going. Just be careful not to do all your running on a treadmill. The repetitive motion without terrain changes due to turns and changing cants can be hard on your legs. They keep repeating exactly the same motions over and over. It's best to mix up running terrains frequently to give your legs some variety. This is good for avoiding injury as well as for fitness.

Cars present a real problem for runners. Running next to traffic is one of the most dangerous things you can do in your triathlon training. Yet every day I see people running in the street with their backs to traffic while wearing a headset to listen to music or the radio. These people must have a death wish! Never run with your back to traffic, and be extra careful when running outdoors with a headset on. When around traffic, be constantly vigilant. Look, listen, and anticipate what drivers might do.

You face many dangerous situations when you run on the streets and roads. One of the most dangerous is approaching an intersection where there is a stopped car waiting for traffic to clear from its left in order to turn right. If you are approaching from the driver's right, chances are good that you will not be seen. Do not enter the intersection until you have made eye contact with the driver or the car has turned. A third option is to cross the intersection by going behind the stopped car. Play it safe when running around traffic.

RUNNING IN HOT WEATHER

There is no greater stress when exercising than heat, especially while running. To control core temperature when it's hot, the body shunts blood to the skin for cooling before returning it to the heart for pumping to the muscles. This means that the heart must work harder during exercise in the heat—not only to fuel the muscles but also to help with cooling—so your pulse rises. When it comes to choosing between running fast and cooling itself, the body will always select cooling first. Sweating helps remove heat through evaporation. And since you sweat more on a hot day, the chance of dehydration increases. Following are some tips to help you prepare for the hot days of summer running, especially if you are doing your first triathlon in the heat:

Acclimate. If you know your first triathlon will be on a hot day, you can help your body get ready. To acclimate to the heat, exercise when the temperature is in the mid-80s or higher for 7 or more days in a 14-day period. Take it very easy during these workouts.

Keep your cool. During a hot workout or race, pour cold water on your head and body to lower your body temperature. Put a little ice in your hat or shirt to help lower body temperature.

Use sunscreen. On a hot, dry day, oil-based sunscreen will block your pores and make conditions worse. Choose a water-based sunscreen instead.

Consider age and heat. Older athletes are more sensitive to the effects of heat than are young athletes. One reason is that sweating tends to decline with aging. Aging competitors also lose more water through urination. The bottom line is that older athletes need to be more scrupulous in taking in fluids.

Take advantage of air-conditioning. Using air-conditioning at night when you sleep will *not* cause you to lose your heat adaptation. If the heat interrupts your sleep pattern, turn the AC on.

Eat for the heat. Contrary to popular opinion, exercising in the heat causes you to burn more calories than exercising in the cold. So

Staying Hydrated

Water deprivation was once the rule in endurance sports. The 1860 Oxford University rowing team was restricted to no more than two pints of fluid daily. In 1909, a widely read book on marathon training advised that runners should not drink during a race: "Don't get in the habit of eating and drinking in a marathon race; some prominent runners do, but it is not beneficial."

In the 1920s and 1930s, one of the top runners of the era, Arthur Newton, wrote, "Even in the warmest English weather, a 26-mile run ought to be manageable with no more than a single drink, or at most two."

As late as 1969, endurance athletes were discouraged from drinking water. Some sports even had rules restricting fluid use. The international governing organization for distance running ruled that "refreshments shall (only) be provided by the organizers of a race after 10 miles, and thereafter every 3 miles. No refreshments may be carried or taken by a competitor other than that provided by the organizers." It wasn't until the 1970s that athletes were encouraged to drink water during workouts and competitions.

More recently, many endurance athletes have become slaves to drinking fluids at regular intervals. Trying to drink to a schedule can be difficult because there are so many factors that will affect your fluid status: the weather, how hard and fast you are running, how cloudy or sunny it is, and how well hydrated you were before starting the workout. But it's easy to stay well hydrated.

To ensure adequate fluid levels, simply drink whenever you are thirsty. For easy exercise lasting less than one hour, water is adequate. For longer workouts sports drinks are recommended.

when adapting nutrition for hot weather, you may need to increase your calories, but only slightly.

Drink for the heat. Be sure to increase your intake of fluids during hot-weather workouts. Drink when you are thirsty. If you do that you'll stay properly hydrated regardless of the environmental conditions. Don't drink just plain water for sessions lasting longer than one hour. Use a sports drink for long runs. The rate of absorption of water when compared with a sports drink is about the same.

Wipe off sweat. Frequently wiping the excess sweat from your face, neck, arms, and other body parts while working out will remove oils and accumulated electrolytes, thus allowing your sweat to be more effective at cooling.

RUNNING EQUIPMENT

Unlike biking, running is an easy sport to get started in. The only gear you really need is running shoes, a decent pair of socks, shorts, and a shirt. Of course, if you go to a running store you will find a lot of accessories, such as hats, water bottle "holsters," special triathlon shoelaces, winter gear, and much more. Some of this, such as winter gear, may be necessary depending on what time of year you're preparing for your first triathlon. But given that getting geared up for the bike can be fairly expensive, I'd suggest purchasing only what you really need for running right now. Here are the basics.

Shoes

Almost all your running budget should be spent on shoes. The cost varies depending on how the shoe is made—what surfaces it is designed for, how lightweight it is, and so forth. Your experience with injuries and soreness should factor into your decision of which shoes to buy. If you've been running for some time, you will probably know what you need. If you are new to running, you can most likely start off with more basic, and less expensive, shoes. In either case, I recommend going to a running specialty store to buy shoes. Other stores may be less expensive, but shoes are so complicated these days that you need someone who knows feet, running, and shoes to help you make the right decision. Some types of shoes, including very expensive ones, could actually cause injuries if they're not a good match for your feet and running style. An experienced salesperson in a running or a triathlon store can guide you through the process by looking at your old shoes (take some old sneakers with you), examining your feet, and watching how you run in different types of shoes.

Most of the shoe companies offer minimalist styles intended to promote good technique. If your previous pair of running shoes had a lot of cushion in the heel cup, you will want to find a shoe that will help you ease into the transition. It takes time to break in a new pair of running shoes, and if the change is drastic it could lead to injury.

Be prepared to spend $75 or more on running shoes. And also understand that they won't last forever. Depending on how big you are, what your running form is like, and what kind of surfaces you run on, expect running shoes to last 300–500 miles. That mileage also includes walking around in them. It's best not to use your running shoes for casual wear; save them for running only. When the first pair begins to get old they can be replaced and become your casual shoes.

Socks

A good pair of socks will have wicking fabrics, mesh weaves, blister prevention, and enhanced durability; these are not your father's gym socks. Again, a running specialty store salesperson can help you match your new shoes with the socks right for you. Expect a pair of good socks to cost at least $6 more than standard socks.

Shirt and Shorts

Running shorts usually have a nylon outer shell and a specially designed brief that wicks moisture away from the skin while allowing airflow for cooling. They often have small pockets for carrying keys, gel packets, sunglasses, or any other small items you may need. Shorts start at about $30.

If you have problems with thigh chafing when running, look for a pair of tight-fitting, thigh-length Lycra shorts to be worn under your running shorts. A lot of triathletes of all sizes and shapes train and race in these shorts exclusively. Some have a small crotch pad built in so they can bike in them too, but I wouldn't recommend doing that except in short races. If chafing during running is all you're trying to prevent, just get a pair of leg-hugging shorts. These may also be appropriate for swimming and will cost about $40 or more.

You can do your runs in a T-shirt when the weather is cool, but on hot days or for long runs, cotton won't hack it because it retains moisture, which can lead to chafing. For these runs a loose-mesh shirt made with a wicking fabric is perfect. These are also sold in running stores and start at about $30.

Women should look for tops with built-in support or purchase a sports bra. Support tops start at about $40, and sports bras at $25. The tops often have a breathable mesh interior panel and a T-strap back with a reflective graphic for visibility in the dark. Many sports bras can be worn without another top.

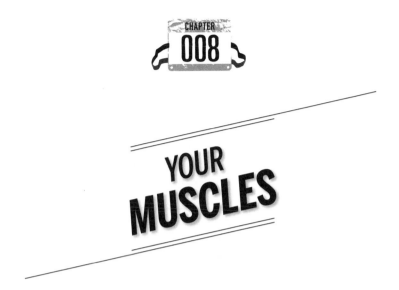

CHAPTER
008

YOUR MUSCLES

Triathlon places a great demand on the aerobic system—your heart, lungs, blood, and aerobic energy pathways. This is the body system we all think of when we prepare for endurance sports such as swimming, biking, and running. Most new triathletes pay little attention to the muscular system, yet it plays a major role in how well you do in a triathlon. Muscles that are strong and supple make it easier to finish on race day. Weak, tight muscles can cause serious problems when tested by hills, strong winds, choppy water, and longer distances.

In the previous three chapters we thoroughly examined swimming, biking, and running. Now we will explore how you can improve your strength and flexibility with weight lifting and stretching.

GETTING STRONGER

Is there a downside to lifting weights? Some endurance athletes don't lift weights out of fear that pumping iron may cause an increase in body weight and slow them down. While younger men can have a tendency to increase muscle mass, it's highly unlikely with the program I've prepared for you. This strength-building program is considerably different than that used by bodybuilders and power lifters. The triathletes I coach have never built so much muscle that they gained weight and became slower; in fact, just the opposite has happened—they have typically become leaner and faster. Building muscle increases the metabolism, which means you burn more calories throughout the day, thus losing excess fat.

Where Do You Find the Time?

One of the biggest challenges you will face in getting ready for your first triathlon is time. How will you find enough not only to swim, bike, and run but also to lift weights and stretch? That's a tall order given how packed your schedule is already. How can you solve this dilemma?

Stretching will fit into your day pretty easily. The ideal time to stretch is the first few minutes right after you swim, bike, or run. But you can also do a little stretching throughout the day at your desk at work, while standing in line at the supermarket, or when watching TV.

Weight lifting, however, is a bigger challenge. The strength exercises at the gym take about 45 minutes to an hour to complete. If you do not have time to go to a gym and you don't have weight equipment at home, there are other options. Most of the exercises in this chapter can be done with elastic resistance bands, which can be purchased at sporting goods stores, through catalogs, and online (www.performbetter.com). In some cases your body weight is enough to facilitate strength improvement. For example, one-leg squats replace leg presses, and push-ups may take the place of bench presses. With a little creativity you can find a way to do most of the gym exercises at home with little or no equipment. Then you can fit strength training into your week more easily. In addition, strength exercises don't have to be done in a single, dedicated workout. You can easily spread them throughout the week, fitting in one or two whenever you have time.

Although research reports mixed results, my experience from coaching hundreds of athletes over 30 years is that lifting weights definitely improves the performance of those who lack power, and this applies especially to those who are new to triathlon. But it appears to be more effective for some sports than for others. For example, it seems to benefit cycling more than running or swimming, although you will improve some in all three sports.

Not all triathletes, or even all cyclists, will see noticeable improvement, however. I find that those most likely to realize a boost in performance are women, older men, and athletes with long, lanky arms and legs. Most males in their 20s and early 30s will probably see less improvement than people over 50.

Time Commitment

The biggest factor in determining whether you should lift weights is how much time you have available to do it. If you just can't find a way to fit even a few more minutes of strength-building exercises into your week once you've done your swim, bike, and run workouts, then strength training must be left out. Triathlon-specific training comes before strength training—you never have to lift weights in a triathlon. That's why in the schedules suggested in Chapter 9 the strength workouts are listed as "optional." Do them if you have time, but otherwise focus on the three sports of triathlon: swimming, biking, and running. But I suspect that it is possible to do some strength building with a little creative thinking about how you use your time.

The most important aspect of this program is consistency. Frequently missing strength workouts negates the reason for doing them. If you know now that you can't get into the gym at least once each week, then don't even start. If this is the case, you probably already have more to do in your life than you can fit in and need to devote your available time to swimming, biking, and running. Getting stronger will make you a better triathlete, but this is not as important as becoming more fit in the three main sports.

Consistency

In setting up a routine, the first issue is how often and on what days you will go to the gym. The schedule in Chapter 9 suggests that you fit in two strength workouts per week for the first seven weeks. If you can only go once, that is still effective. You'll see some improvement over time if you're consistent, although not as much as if you worked on strength twice every week. The two days are best separated by 72–96 hours. So, for example, one gym session on Monday and another on Thursday or Friday is just right. If you do the workouts within a three-day time frame, there will be a big gap until the next gym workout the following week. That gap will make the workouts slightly less effective.

Where to Work Out

Another thing to consider is where you will do the strength-building workouts. I have been referring to the gym, but that may not be an option for you. If you have some strength equipment at home, you can do it there. That may even save you time. Almost every exercise in this chapter can be done with stretch bands also. These are basically large rubber bands and can be purchased at sporting goods stores, online, or from catalogs.

Doubling Up

A lot of triathletes swim at their gym's pool, so they do swim and weight workouts on the same day, one right after the other. This saves time spent driving back and forth. If you do that, make the swim workout the first session each time. It's not a good idea to swim with muscles fatigued from weight lifting; that will cause you to build bad swim habits. If you must do one of the sports right *after* lifting weights, it's best to make that cycling, as running on tired legs can easily lead to injury.

My strength program will give you nice results within a minimal time commitment, which basically means your first triathlon will be easier than it might otherwise have been. I've used this program with lots of other triathlon newbies—and with great success. I am confident that it will work for you too.

You won't be lifting heavy weights because your muscles will be getting a lot of work already with the other sports, and we don't want to risk injury from overuse. Instead, you will first learn to do the exercises correctly with light weights. After improving your weight-lifting skills, we'll make the loads a little heavier to begin building strength.

STRENGTH EXERCISES

One of the most important parts of any strength program is deciding which exercises you will do. There are lots of exercises you could do at the gym to get stronger, but your focus should be only on getting stronger for triathlon. You won't win a bodybuilding contest on this program, but I expect that is okay with you.

It's important that the resistance exercises you do match the movements of the sport for which you are training. For example, there is little reason for a swimmer to do leg presses, but this is a quite valuable exercise for cyclists since the movement is similar to pedaling a bike. The exercises shown later in this chapter are based on the movements of triathlon and closely mimic them in order to make your triathlon muscles stronger. Also, some of the exercises here are necessary to help correct muscular imbalances, which may lead to frequent injury.

It's best that the strength exercises involve more than one joint ("multi-joint") whenever possible. For example, a seated knee extension is a single-joint exercise because only one joint—the knee—is used (see Figure 8.11). The leg press (see Figure 8.1), however, is a multi-joint exercise involving the hip, knee, and ankle. Multi-joint exercises more closely mimic the movements of triathlon, and they save time in the weight room because larger parts of the body and more muscles can be worked with each exercise. Single-joint exercises are used here to isolate muscles prone to triathlon injury.

The first exercise listed for each muscle group is what you should do if you have gym equipment available. If you do not, use the following exercise(s) in each section. These alternative exercises are designed to be done at home with an elastic resistance band or your body weight. There is no reason to do both of the variations.

1 LEG-BUILDING EXERCISES

Leg Press (FIGURE 8.1)

Improves pedaling strength for cycling and hill running power.

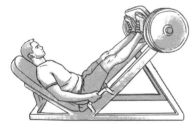

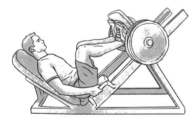

FIGURE 8.1

1. Center your feet on the middle portion of the platform about 10–12 inches apart, center to center. Your feet should be parallel, not angled out, and in the middle of the platform.
2. Press the platform up until your legs are almost straight, with your knees just short of locking out.
3. Lower the platform until your knees are about 8 inches from your chest, no lower. This should create about a 90-degree angle in your knees. (It may help to have a friend check your knee angle to make sure it is about 90 degrees.) Keep your knees in line with your feet throughout the movement—don't let them flare out wide or collapse toward each other.
4. Return to the start position and repeat.

Resistance Band Squat (FIGURE 8.2)

Both this exercise and the one-leg squat may be used to build greater ankle, knee, and hip strength, which helps to improve turning the pedals and running powerfully.

1. Holding the ends of a couple of yards of resistance band, stand with your feet on the middle of the band and about 10–12 inches apart.
2. Squat until your knees are at a 90-degree bend. Keep your back straight, rear end low, and head up. Stretch the band to increase the tension.
3. Return to the start position and repeat.

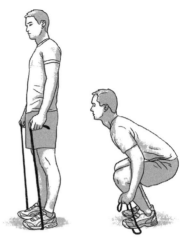

FIGURE 8.2

One-Leg Squat (FIGURE 8.3)

1. Stand on one leg with the other bent at the knee. Place one hand against a wall to stabilize yourself.
2. Keeping your head up and back straight, bend the support leg to lower yourself until that knee is at a 90-degree angle (have someone help you get this right).
3. Stand back up. Complete all the repetitions with one leg before doing the other in the same manner.

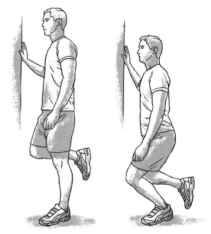

FIGURE 8.3

2 BACK-BUILDING EXERCISES

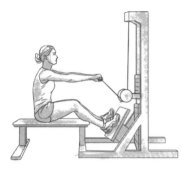

FIGURE 8.4

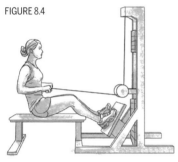

Seated Row (FIGURE 8.4)

Simulates the movement of pulling on the handlebars while climbing a hill on a bicycle in a seated position. Strengthens the core—lower and upper back.

1. Grasp the bar with your arms fully extended and your hands about 10–12 inches apart. Your back should be straight.
2. Pull the bar toward your lower chest, keeping your elbows close to your body. Minimize movement at the waist by using your back muscles to stabilize your position.
3. Return to the start position and repeat.

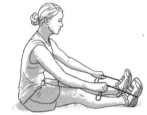

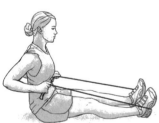

FIGURE 8.5

Seated Row with Resistance Band (FIGURE 8.5)

1. Sit on the floor with your legs out in front of you and your back straight.
2. While holding each end of the resistance band, loop it under your feet.
3. Bend forward at the waist, keeping your back straight, and stretch the band until it is tight.
4. With a small rowing motion, pull the ends of the band to the sides of your lower chest.
5. Return to the start position and repeat.

3 CHEST-BUILDING EXERCISES

Chest Press (FIGURE 8.6)

Stabilizes the shoulders for swimming and strengthens the shoulder girdle and triceps. Can be done with free weights or on a machine.

1. Grasp the bar with your hands just slightly farther apart than the width of your shoulders.
2. Slowly lower the bar to your chest.
3. Return to the start position and repeat.

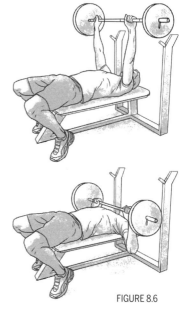

Push-Up (FIGURE 8.7)

As with the chest press, this exercise stabilizes the shoulders for swimming and strengthens the shoulder girdle and triceps. Either the toes or the knees can be used as support points. To increase the difficulty, use an unstable surface such as a stability ball under the feet, or disc pillows under the hands.

1. From the support position with the arms fully extended, slowly lower your chest to the floor.
2. Maintain a straight back with your head in the same plane as your spine without allowing either the spine or the head to sag.
3. When your chest is within 2–3 inches of the floor, slowly push up until you return to the starting position while still maintaining good posture. Repeat.

FIGURE 8.6

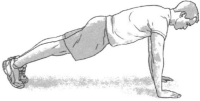

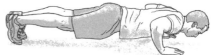

FIGURE 8.7

I call exercises 4, 5, and 6 "personal weakness" exercises. The idea here is to do only one of these three based on which area of your legs gives you the most trouble, in order to make it stronger. If it is your calves and Achilles tendon (shin splints, sore calves, Achilles tendinitis), then do exercise 4. If your weakness is the muscles and tendons around your knees (cramping or general soreness in the muscles and tendons around your knees), then do exercise 5. And if your weakness is the hamstrings on the back of your upper leg (soreness, tightness, muscle pulls), do exercise 6. If you have more than one such personal weakness area, then do two or all three of these exercises. You may also need to do a lot of stretching for this personal weakness area. That's covered later in this chapter.

4 CALF-BUILDING EXERCISES

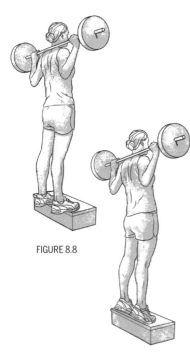

FIGURE 8.8

Heel Raise (FIGURE 8.8)

If you have experienced calf or Achilles tendon injuries, this exercise may help strengthen those tissues. It also improves lower leg strength for running.

1. Stand with the balls of your feet on a 1- to 2-inch riser such as a board, with your heels on the floor and a barbell on your shoulders or a dumbbell in each hand.
2. Point your feet straight ahead, about shoulder width apart.
3. Raise up on your toes.
4. Return to the start position and repeat.

Resistance Band
Toe Raises (FIGURE 8.9)

Assume the same position as in steps
1 and 2 of the heel raise exercise, only with
a resistance band under the balls of your
feet and the ends of it in each hand, with
your arms straight down at your sides.

1. Rise up on your toes. Shorten the
   resistance band to increase the load.
2. Return to the start position and
   repeat.

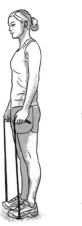
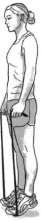

FIGURE 8.9

5   KNEE-STRENGTHENING EXERCISES

Knee Extension (FIGURE 8.10)

This exercise may help those with past knee
problems by balancing the strength between
the medial and the lateral quadriceps. If you
have a history of knee problems, check with
your doctor to ensure that this is the correct
exercise for you.

1. Start with your knees fully extended and
   toes pointing slightly to the outside.
2. Lower the weight only about 8 inches
   (do not go all the way down—you may be
   able to lock the machine out to prevent
   your foot from going too low).
3. Return to the start position and repeat.

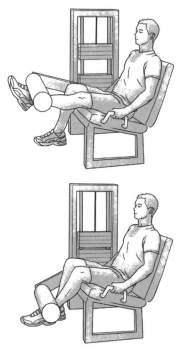

FIGURE 8.10

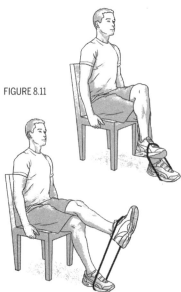

FIGURE 8.11

Knee Extension with Resistance Band (FIGURE 8.11)

The knee-extension is difficult to simulate at home, but here is one alternative.

1. Sit in a straight-backed chair with your legs crossed so that your left knee is resting on your right leg.
2. Loop a resistance band over your left ankle and under your right foot.
3. Straighten your left knee, raising your lower leg to the horizontal position.
4. Lower it and repeat. Shorten the resistance band to increase the tension.

6   HAMSTRING-BUILDING EXERCISES

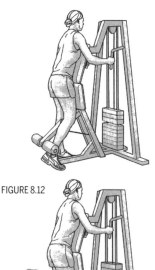

FIGURE 8.12

Leg Curl (FIGURE 8.12)

By strengthening the hamstrings on the back of the upper leg, the balance of strength between that muscle and the larger quadriceps on the front of the thigh is improved. This may help prevent hamstring injuries in athletes who are plagued by this problem. Leg curl machines are used either standing (shown here), seated, or on the stomach.

1. Pull your foot toward your rear end until your knee is at about a 90-degree angle (have someone help you get this right). Don't allow your rear end to arch upward.
2. Return to the start position and repeat.

Assisted Leg Curl (FIGURE 8.13)

You'll need a helper for this one.

1. Lie on your stomach on the floor with your helper at your feet.

2. Have the helper hold on to the heel of one foot as you pull it toward your rear end. The helper should provide just enough resistance to make the foot move up slowly.

3. Return to the start position and repeat.

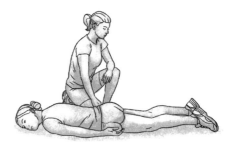
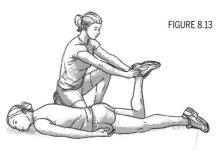

FIGURE 8.13

7   ABDOMINAL-BUILDING EXERCISES

Abdominal with Twist (FIGURE 8.14)

This is a basic core exercise to help stabilize your body while swimming, biking, and running.

1. Sit on a decline board with your knees bent at about a 90-degree angle.

2. Cross your arms over your chest. Holding a weight plate against your chest is optional. (Do not pull on your head or neck.)

3. Lower your body to about a 45-degree angle to the floor.

4. Return to the start position with a twist of your upper body. With each repetition, alternate twisting to the right and the left as you rise up.

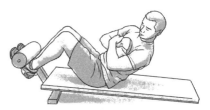
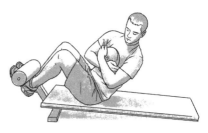

FIGURE 8.14

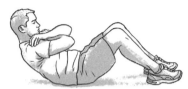
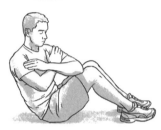

Crunches with Twist (FIGURE 8.15)

Crunches help to improve core strength for better posture and transfer of power to the water,
pedals, or ground.

1. On the floor, sit with your knees bent at
   about a 90-degree angle and cross your
   arms over your chest.
2. Curl up. Alternate touching your right elbow
   to your left leg and your left elbow to your
   right leg.

FIGURE 8.15

8   SHOULDER-BUILDING EXERCISES

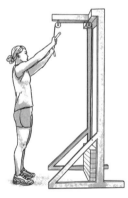

Standing, Bent-Arm
Lat Pull Down (FIGURE 8.16)

This increases the strength of your shoulders
to make swimming easier.

1. While standing (or on your knees) at the lat
   pull-down station, position the bar so it is a
   few inches above your head.
2. Place your hands on top of the bar about
   shoulder width apart, with your elbows
   slightly bent.
3. Maintain a high elbow position and push the
   bar down by rotating your shoulders until
   the bar is at chest level.
4. Return to the start position and repeat.

FIGURE 8.16

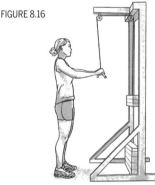

Resistance Band
Lat Pull (FIGURE 8.17)

Open a door and stand facing the edge
of it so that you can have one arm on
either side.

1. Place your resistance band over the top
   of the door so that it hangs down
   on both sides.

2. Grasp both ends of the band and,
   maintaining a high elbow position, pull
   down by rotating your shoulder until
   the bands are at chest level.

3. Return to the start position and repeat.

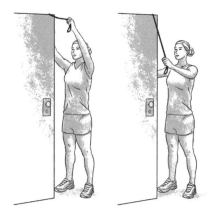

FIGURE 8.17

How Much Weight to Use

Before you begin your strength workouts, you need to figure out how much
weight to lift. Weight lifters refer to "repetition max," or "RM." This is how
much weight someone can lift a given number of times. For example, if you
can leg press 200 pounds 15 times, your 15RM is 200.

As you start this program to build your strength, you will be lifting 30RM
loads, which is quite light. In fact, even though you can lift the load 30 times,
you will stop at 20 repetitions the first few sessions you are in the gym
because you want to become good at doing the exercises before progressing.
That will take perhaps four strength sessions. After that you will increase the
loads to 15RM and do 12–15 repetitions. To be on the safe side and to reduce
the possibility of lost swim, bike, and run training due to sore muscles, it's
best to stop each exercise when you feel as if you could do only one or two
more reps. Do not push to the point of failure—meaning you can't complete
even one more rep—on any exercise. You may still get a little soreness, but it
will go away more quickly than if you lifted to failure.

CONTINUED

CONTINUED

So how do you decide what your 30RM or 15RM is? The only sure way is to test yourself by seeing how many reps you can do with given loads. This isn't the best approach for endurance athletes because it always makes them sore for several days afterward. I think you can probably guess your loads based on what you discover in the first few gym sessions. You don't have to be precise, but you do need to challenge yourself a bit every few days. Try increasing the load by 5 percent every third or fourth session to see if you can handle it. If you are progressing normally, you should see a steady improvement in strength in the first few weeks.

STRENGTH-TRAINING PHASES

In the next chapter you will learn about *periodization*, which organizes your training to improve fitness. This is basically a way of systematically scheduling variety into your training program so that you are race-ready when you get to your first triathlon. Your strength training is a part of this scheduling process, so you will vary the workouts a bit every few weeks. This variety is based on different periods, or "phases," of strength training, each of which has a specific purpose.

You will progress through three phases of strength training in the 12 weeks leading up to your first triathlon: *anatomical adaptation* (AA), *maximum transition* (MT), and *strength maintenance* (SM). Each phase lasts a few weeks, just enough time to accomplish its purpose. Table 8.1 summarizes all the details of your strength training in one place. This same pattern is built into your 12-week training plan in Chapter 9.

Here are the three phases of your strength-training program.

Anatomical Adaptation (AA)

The purpose of anatomical adaptation is to prepare the muscles and tendons for the heavier work of the MT phase and to perfect the movements of each exercise. More exercises are done in this phase than in the other two because the goal is to improve overall strength. In AA you do three sets of each exercise. A "set" is a number of repetitions of a given exercise. In AA the first 20 reps are done to completion, then you stop to rest. Complete the other two sets before you move on to the next exercise and perform three sets of it. The loads are very light, allowing for a high number of reps (20). You could do more than 20 reps, but don't, because what you want to accomplish with this workout is perfection of technique. Doing more will cause fatigue, resulting in sloppy technique. After four of these workouts in two weeks, you will begin to notice that you are already getting stronger.

Maximum Transition (MT)

This is really the heart of your strength-building program for this 12-week period. If you felt as if you were getting stronger in AA, you'll notice an even bigger change after eight of these workouts. The number of exercises is pared back a bit so you can focus on getting stronger in the most triathlon-specific areas (these are listed for each week in the training plan in Chapter 9). The loads increase the first week to 20RM, and you do 15–20 reps. These two sessions are a transition period, allowing you to adjust to heavier loads and make sure you are getting the weight right. During the next three weeks the loads are increased to 15RM, and you do 10–15 reps. Stop each set when you feel that you can do only one or two more reps. The number of reps you can complete on a given day may vary depending on how tired you are from your swim, bike, and run workouts. Don't let that bother you; it's normal.

Strength Maintenance (SM)

The purpose of SM is to maintain the strength you've built in the previous weeks of the MT phase. It takes only about half as much work to maintain a given level of fitness as it took to achieve it. That means you can maintain your strength once you have thoroughly developed it by only lifting weights once per week instead of twice. It also means that you have to do only one heavy set of each exercise to stay strong.

In SM, when you do strength exercises one day a week, you will do one light set (20RM) to warm up, followed by one heavy set (15RM) to maintain strength. For both sets you will do 10–15 reps. This means the warm-up set will be quite easy and the heavy set quite hard. This will keep you strong for the next several weeks.

Table 8.1 Strength Training at a Glance

	WEEKS TO TRI	WORKOUTS/ WEEK	EXERCISES	LOAD	SETS	REPS
ANATOMICAL ADAPTATION	12	2	1, 2, 3 (4, 5, or 6), 7, 8	30RM	3	20
	11	2	1, 2, 3 (4, 5, or 6), 7, 8	30RM	3	20
MAXIMUM TRANSITION	10	2	1, 2 (4, 5, or 6), 7, 8	20RM	3	15–20
	9	2	1, 2 (4, 5, or 6), 7, 8	15RM	3	10–15
	8	2	1, 2 (4, 5, or 6), 7, 8	15RM	3	10–15
	7	2	1, 2 (4, 5, or 6), 7, 8	15RM	3	10–15
STRENGTH MAINTENANCE	6	1	1, 2 (4, 5, or 6), 7, 8	20, 15RM	2	10–15
	5	1	1, 2 (4, 5, or 6), 7, 8	20, 15RM	2	10–15
	4	1	1, 2 (4, 5, or 6), 7, 8	20, 15RM	2	10–15
	3	1	1, 2 (4, 5, or 6), 7, 8	20, 15RM	2	10–15
	2	1	1, 2 (4, 5, or 6), 7, 8	20, 15RM	2	10–15
	—	1	0	—	—	—

Note: RM = repetition max

You don't need to memorize Table 8.1 and these explanations because this routine is built into your training plan in Chapter 9. They are included here so you can see the details of what you will be doing in the coming weeks and understand the different goals of each phase.

IMPROVING YOUR FLEXIBILITY

Some people are naturally flexible. They can put their palms on the floor easily in a forward fold, touch their fingers behind their shoulder blades, squat without falling backward, and sit on the floor with their legs spread apart, touching their nose to their knees. Most of us aren't so flexibly endowed. If you're naturally tight, you need to become more flexible. If you are already "loose as a goose" in all your joints, then you need not spend much time stretching. However, it's rare to find such total-body flexibility. It's far more likely that someone who has flexible shoulders is tight in the hips or some other area. It's been my experience that practically every triathlete benefits from stretching several times a week.

Of the three sports, swimming requires the most flexibility, especially in the shoulders and ankles. If your shoulders are tight, you'll have a hard time getting your elbow above your hand on the recovery part of the stroke, creating an inefficient zigzag swim technique. People with tight ankles who are new to swimming often go backward when they use a kickboard. If your hamstrings are tight, you are more prone to experiencing cycling and running injuries. Tight, inflexible hamstrings also contribute to low back problems, which are at epidemic proportions in North America. Enthusiastic triathletes often find that the demands of the individual sports can lead to new areas of tightness. For example, lots of cycling can make your quads (thighs) tight, and running contributes to tight calf muscles (and thus shin pain) for newbies.

If you can identify areas of tightness, a little time spent stretching every day prevents soreness and injury and makes you a better triathlete. Prevention is always more comfortable, less time-consuming, and cheaper than medical treatment.

Stretching Exercises

There are as many different ways to stretch as there are types of bicycles. And just like bikes, each kind of stretching has unique advantages and disadvantages. This creates a lot of confusion. You will use the easiest and most common form of stretching—*static stretching*.

Static stretching has been around since the 1970s and is still the most widely used method by triathletes. It's really quite simple. Take a position that stretches a given muscle group and hold it for several seconds. You may find that some tight muscles feel best when stretched this way for 15–20 seconds. For others 8–12 seconds feels right. The key to static stretching is not so much how long you hold the position, but how frequently you stretch.

A few seconds spent stretching different muscles throughout the day will greatly improve your flexibility over time. Good times to stretch are before and after workouts and at the end of your day just before bed. Each of these may take only five minutes or so. It's also easy to fit little stretches, such as shin stretching by pointing your toes, into your day when sitting at your desk, standing in line at the checkout, or riding in a car.

Although stretching does not have to follow a specific routine, there are a few stretches that will directly aid your swimming, biking, and running. The exercises I've included here are most effective after workouts. Feel free to incorporate the other stretches that you've found to be beneficial.

Shoulder Reach (FIGURE 8.18)

This is a great exercise to do before and after swimming to improve the flexibility of your shoulders.

1. Extend your arms over your head and cross one wrist over the other while interlocking your hands.
2. With your elbows behind your ears, straighten your arms and reach up.

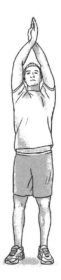

FIGURE 8.18

Ankle Sit (FIGURE 8.19)

Another swimming exercise, this sit will loosen tight ankles, allowing you to be more streamlined in the water.

1. Sit on your shins on a padded surface or folded towel with your toes pointed (not splayed to the sides).
2. Sit on your heels.
3. Lean backward slightly until you feel an easy stretch.

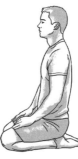

FIGURE 8.19

Twister (FIGURE 8.20)

This exercise will help you become more flexible in the shoulders, allowing your arm recovery movement in swimming to be much easier.

1. With your back facing a wall, grasp a stationary object at about shoulder height.
2. Look away from the arm being stretched and simultaneously twist your body away from it.

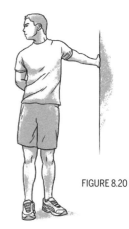

FIGURE 8.20

Stork Stand (FIGURE 8.21)

This exercise works well for both biking and running, but it is especially beneficial before and after a bike ride.

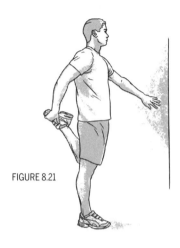

FIGURE 8.21

1. While balancing against your bike or a wall, grasp your right foot behind your back with your left hand. Note that you're using the opposite hand and foot.
2. Gently pull up and away from your rear end with your hand while keeping the bent knee even with or behind the straight knee.
3. Keep your head up and stand tall—do not bend over at the waist.

Triangle (FIGURE 8.22)

Stretching the hamstrings this way is beneficial to both running and biking.

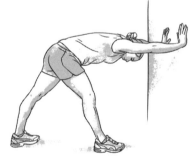

FIGURE 8.22

1. Bend over at the waist while leaning on your bike or a wall.
2. Place the leg to be stretched forward, with your foot about 18 inches from the bike or wall.
3. Keep the other leg directly behind the first. The farther back this leg is placed, the greater the stretch.
4. With your weight on the front foot, sag your upper body toward the floor. You should feel the stretch in the hamstring (back of the thigh) of your forward leg.

Pull Down (FIGURE 8.23)

This is especially good for shoulder flexibility for swimming, but this exercise also relieves tightness due to biking and running.

1. Hold on to your bike or a railing for balance, with your weight resting on your arms.
2. Allow your head to sag deeply between your outstretched arms to create a stretch in your lats (sides of the torso).

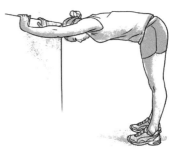

FIGURE 8.23

Squat (FIGURE 8.24)

The squat is a great lower back and leg stretch for running and biking. If you don't have time for any other stretches, this is the one to do.

1. Hold on to something for balance and squat down, keeping your heels on the floor (this is easier with your bike shoes off).
2. Allow your rear end to sag close to your heels as you rock forward.

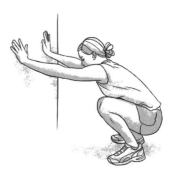

FIGURE 8.24

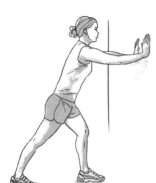

FIGURE 8.25

Wall Lean (FIGURE 8.25)

This is probably the most popular running stretch of all time. It helps loosen up tight calf muscles.

1. Lean against a wall, with the leg to be stretched straight behind you and the other leg forward, supporting most of your weight.
2. Keep the heel of the rear foot on the floor as you lean, with the toes pointed straight ahead. The farther forward your hips move, the greater the stretch on your calf. Elbows can be straight or bent.
3. There are two major calf muscles. To stretch the other one, bend your rear knee.

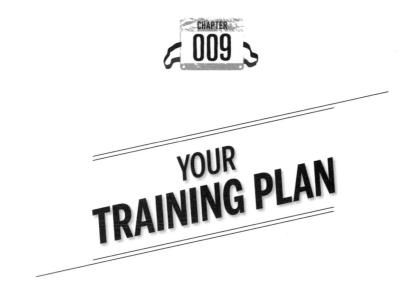

YOUR TRAINING PLAN

Are you feeling overwhelmed yet? There is so much to learn about the sport of triathlon that it can leave you feeling a bit underwater. But don't worry; everyone goes through this.

Training in one sport, such as running, is hard enough. Training in three sports at the same time is more than three times as challenging in part because you need to blend so many different workouts into a week. When preparing for a triathlon you obviously can't do as much swimming as a swimmer does. The same goes for cycling and running. An athlete in any of these individual sports will put in far more training time and distance than the typical triathlete does. For example, the average beginner athlete in each of these sports probably exercises about five to six hours each week. If you tried to match the training of a swimmer, cyclist, or runner, you'd have to exercise 15–18 hours a week, and that does not include strength training. Obviously that is not going to happen.

Assuming you have about three to four hours each week to work out, you need to figure out how to make the best use of that time so your fitness improves steadily. If you overdo it you may easily become overtrained, injured, or sick. But if you do too little your fitness won't improve enough to finish your first triathlon. This is the quandary every new triathlete faces.

In this chapter I will help you solve this problem by providing a training plan you can follow and modify as necessary. It's not possible to have a one-schedule-fits-all training plan; there are just too many variables, such as time available to exercise, prior experience in one or more sports, how quickly one recovers, and individual rates of fitness improvement. So I've designed this training plan with optional workouts based on your unique situation.

Why should you even have a plan? Why not just swim, bike, run, and do strength workouts when you have the time? That may work for a few people, but chances are it won't work for you. I expect you are like most triathletes—very busy, with too much to do already. And yet somehow you are going to try to wedge triathlon training into each day. Without a plan of what you will do every day, you likely won't do much. A well-defined plan keeps you on schedule to achieve your goal. I have made your plan as user-friendly and flexible as possible so you can stay on track.

Before we get down to the nuts and bolts of a training plan, let's review a few basic concepts on how to get fit.

GETTING FIT: THE BIG PICTURE

While training for your first triathlon, there are only four things you can change to improve fitness.

> *Mode:* This is the type of workout you do—swim, bike, or run. Of course, strength and stretching exercises are also modes of exercise.
> *Frequency:* This is how often you train. If you exercise once each day, your frequency is seven per week.
> *Duration:* This is how long your workouts are, either in time or distance. Combining duration (how long) with frequency (how often) gives you "volume"—how much total training you do for a given pe-

riod of time, such as a week. When a triathlete says she trained six hours this week, she is talking about both duration and frequency.

Intensity: This is how hard or easy your exercise is. (Later in this chapter I discuss the Rating of Perceived Exertion scale, the easiest measure of workout intensity. Chapter 10 will introduce other devices such as heart rate monitors and power meters, which measure intensity in a more precise manner.)

Although mode, duration, and frequency are easy to measure and talk about, it can be difficult to arrive at the perfect balance that allows you to be ready and adequately recovered for race day.

The plan I've put together for you in this chapter is based on a system of training called periodization. As mentioned in Chapter 8, this is really nothing more than a way of organizing training so that you train hard when you need to, rest when you need to, and are race-fit the day of your triathlon. Using periodization, your weekly hours of training will increase steadily as your conditioning improves and you are able to handle more. Essentially, your workouts will become progressively longer.

They will also become more like the particular event you are training for, requiring more effort over time. If there are going to be hills on the course, eventually you will need to include hills in your workouts. If the triathlon you chose is held at the height of the summer heat, you will need to practice training in the higher temperatures as you get closer to race day. All this is called training specificity—your workouts will become increasingly more like the race over time.

The most important aspect of preparation for your first triathlon is consistency. There's no doubt that you will miss some workouts, but you can't miss many. Occasionally there will be days when something pops up in your life and prevents you from getting on your bike right after work as you had planned, such as the boss asking you to work overtime. There will be some Saturday when taking the kids out of town to a soccer game will be more important. You may catch a flu bug and miss a few days of training. It's important to keep such interruptions to your training plan to a minimum. If missing workouts becomes a weekly occurrence, your chances of achieving your triathlon goal will be greatly diminished.

Experienced triathletes have developed coping strategies for these interruptions to training. Seasoned triathletes will run during their lunch break on days they need to work late. They will get up earlier to work out on mornings when their kid has a soccer game. They will watch the big game on TV while riding a stationary bike rather than missing either the game or the ride. To get in shape for your first triathlon, you will have to become a master at such coping strategies. If you allow life to get in the way of your workouts too often, you just won't be ready.

FINDING THE RIGHT TRAINING PLAN

Four plans are offered here for a sprint-distance and for an Olympic-distance triathlon to help you organize your training. You might not need to use them if you already have a good idea of how to prepare yourself for your first triathlon. These plans allow 12 weeks for you to get in shape. If you're starting from ground zero, that should be just about right. If you have been working out for a few weeks, you can jump in at a level that closely matches what you are doing now.

The beginner plans (Tables 9.1 and 9.5) are for the person who is brand new to all three sports. These will help you gradually build fitness in swimming, biking, and running. The swimmer plans (Tables 9.2 and 9.6) are intended for the person who has a good background in that sport and usually works out with a masters swim group. If you're an accomplished swimmer who trains alone, then simply plug in your own swim workouts on the days calling for a masters swim. The cyclist plans (Tables 9.3 and 9.7) offer much harder and longer bike workouts for the experienced and fit bike rider. If this describes you, I have a suggestion. Many serious cyclists do most of their riding with groups in mini-races. You should avoid these when training for a triathlon because the recovery "cost" is just too high and will cut into your swim and run training. The runner plans (Tables 9.4 and 9.8) are for the person who has a running background and has built up considerable fitness in this sport. The running workouts here are much more challenging than in the other three plans.

If you were once a swimmer, cyclist, or runner but have been out of training for some time, it's probably best to start with the beginner plan and modify the workouts in your former sport as you progress. Your fitness in that sport may well come back faster than for the other sports. At that point you may even decide to switch over to the more advanced plan for your former sport.

Common features of the plans are described below.

Workout Descriptions

The plans refer to workouts by number, such as "Bike #2." Each workout description can be found in the appropriate appendix. The swim workouts are in Appendix B, the bike workouts in Appendix C, the run workouts in Appendix D, the combination workouts in Appendix E, and the strength workouts in Appendix F. Use the thumb tabs to find these sections quickly as you become more familiar with this book.

Workout Intensity

Each of the workouts in the appendixes tells you how hard to exercise by using the Rating of Perceived Exertion (RPE) scale:

Zone 1   Very easy with light breathing

Zone 2   Easy with increased breathing

Zone 3   Moderately hard with somewhat labored breathing

Zone 4   Hard with labored breathing

Zone 5   Very hard, very difficult to breathe

This scale may be used for all sports, but it is the only one used for swim workouts. For bike and run workouts, if you are using a heart rate monitor, refer to your heart rate training zones, which you can calculate by using the method shown on pages 163–164 in Chapter 10. But you don't have to use a heart rate monitor; RPE is fine.

Table 9.1 Sprint Beginner Plan

WEEKS TO TRI	MONDAY	TUESDAY	WEDNESDAY	
12	Optional strength #1 or day off	Swim #1 and optional run #1	Bike #1	
11	Optional strength #1 or day off	Swim #1 and optional run #1	Bike #2	
10	Optional strength #2 or day off	Swim #2 and optional run #2	Bike #1	
9 R&R	Optional strength #3 or day off	Swim #2 and optional run #3	Bike #5	
8	Optional strength #3 or day off	Swim #3 and optional run #8	Bike #1	
7	Optional strength #3 or day off	Swim #3 and optional run #4	Bike #7	
6 R&R	Optional strength #4 or day off	Swim #4 and optional run #8	Bike #7	
5	Optional strength #4 or day off	Swim #4 and optional run #4	Bike #9	
4	Optional strength #4 or day off	Swim #5 and optional run #8	Bike #8	
3 R&R	Optional strength #4 or day off	Swim #5 and optional run #8	Bike #8	
2	Optional strength #4 or day off	Swim #5 and optional run #4	Bike #9	
1 Saturday Race	Day off	Bike #3	Run #1	
1 Sunday Race	Day off	Swim #5	Bike #3	

Note: Workout details for the swim, bike, run, combination, and strength workouts are in Appendix A. If you don't have access to a gym, replace all strength workouts with resistance exercises, also found in Appendix A.

Sprint Plan

THURSDAY	FRIDAY	SATURDAY	SUNDAY
Run #8 and optional strength #1	Swim #1 and optional bike #1	Bike #2	Run #1 and optional swim #1
Run #8 and optional strength #1	Swim #1 and optional bike #1	Bike #3	Run #2 and optional swim #1
Run #8 and optional strength #2	Swim #2 and optional bike #3	Bike #4	Run #3 and optional swim #1
Run #8 and optional strength #3	Swim #2 and optional bike #3	Bike #9	Run #4 and optional swim #1
Run #3 and optional strength #3	Swim #3 and optional bike #1	Bike #9	Run #4 and optional swim #1
Run #8 and optional strength #3	Swim #3 and optional bike #3	Bike #10	Run #5 and optional swim #1
Run #4	Swim #4 and optional bike #3	Run #5	Combination #1 and optional swim #1
Run #8	Swim #4 and optional bike #2	Run #6	Combination #2 and optional swim #1
Run #6	Swim #6 and optional bike #3	Bike #9 and optional swim #1	Swim #6 and combination #3
Run #7	Swim #6 and optional bike #3	Bike #3 and optional swim #1	Swim #6 and combination #4
Run #8	Swim #6 and optional bike #1	Bike #1 and optional swim #1	Swim #6 and combination #3
Swim #2	Bike #1	*YOUR FIRST TRIATHLON*	Day off
Run #1	Swim #2	Bike #1	*YOUR FIRST TRIATHLON*

Sprint Plan

Table 9.2 Sprint Experienced Swimmer Plan

WEEKS TO TRI	MONDAY	TUESDAY	WEDNESDAY	
12	Optional strength #1 or day off	Swim #7 and optional run #1	Bike #1	
11	Optional strength #1 or day off	Swim #7 and optional run #1	Bike #2	
10	Optional strength #2 or day off	Swim #7 and optional run #2	Bike #1	
9 R&R	Optional strength #3 or day off	Swim #7 and optional run #3	Bike #5	
8	Optional strength #3 or day off	Swim #7 and optional run #8	Bike #1	
7	Optional strength #3 or day off	Swim #7 and optional run #4	Bike #7	
6 R&R	Optional strength #4 or day off	Swim #7 and optional run #8	Bike #7	
5	Optional strength #4 or day off	Swim #7 and optional run #4	Bike #9	
4	Optional strength #4 or day off	Swim #7 and optional run #8	Bike #8	
3 R&R	Optional strength #4 or day off	Swim #7 and optional run #8	Bike #8	
2	Optional strength #4 or day off	Swim #7 and optional run #4	Bike #9	
1 Saturday Race	Day off	Bike #3	Run #1	
1 Sunday Race	Day off	Swim #5	Bike #3	

Note: Workout details for the swim, bike, run, combination, and strength workouts are in Appendix A. If you don't have access to a gym, replace all strength workouts with resistance exercises, also found in Appendix A.

Sprint Plan

THURSDAY	FRIDAY	SATURDAY	SUNDAY
Run #8 and optional strength #1	Swim #7 and optional bike #1	Bike #2	Run #1 and optional swim #8
Run #8 and optional strength #1	Swim #7 and optional bike #1	Bike #3	Run #2 and optional swim #8
Run #8 and optional strength #2	Swim #7 and optional bike #3	Bike #4	Run #3 and optional swim #8
Run #8 and optional strength #3	Swim #7 and optional bike #3	Bike #9	Run #4 and optional swim #8
Run #3 and optional strength #3	Swim #7 and optional bike #1	Bike #9	Run #4 and optional swim #8
Run #8 and optional strength #3	Swim #7 and optional bike #3	Bike #10	Run #5 and optional swim #8
Run #4	Swim #7 and optional bike #3	Run #5	Combination #1 and optional swim #8
Run #8	Swim #7 and optional bike #3	Run #6	Combination #2 and optional swim #8
Run #6	Swim #7 and optional bike #3	Bike #9 and optional swim #8	Swim #6 and combination #3
Run #7	Swim #7 and optional bike #3	Bike #3 and optional swim #8	Swim #6 and combination #4
Run #8	Swim #7 and optional bike #1	Bike #1 and optional swim #8	Swim #6 and combination #3
Swim #2	Bike #1	*YOUR FIRST TRIATHLON*	Day off
Run #1	Swim #4	Bike #1	*YOUR FIRST TRIATHLON*

Table 9.3 Sprint Experienced Cyclist Plan

Sprint Plan

WEEKS TO TRI	MONDAY	TUESDAY	WEDNESDAY	
12	Optional strength #1 or day off	Swim #1 and optional run #1	Bike #8	
11	Optional strength #1 or day off	Swim #1 and optional run #1	Bike #8	
10	Optional strength #2 or day off	Swim #2 and optional run #2	Bike #8	
9 R&R	Optional strength #3 or day off	Swim #2 and optional run #3	Bike #8	
8	Optional strength #3 or day off	Swim #3 and optional run #8	Bike #10	
7	Optional strength #3 or day off	Swim #3 and optional run #4	Bike #15	
6 R&R	Optional strength #4 or day off	Swim #4 and optional run #8	Bike #15	
5	Optional strength #4 or day off	Swim #4 and optional run #4	Bike #10	
4	Optional strength #4 or day off	Swim #5 and optional run #8	Bike #15	
3 R&R	Optional strength #4 or day off	Swim #5 and optional run #8	Bike #15	
2	Optional strength #4 or day off	Swim #5 and optional run #4	Bike #10	
1 Saturday Race	Day off	Bike #4	Run #1	
1 Sunday Race	Day off	Swim #5	Bike #4	

Note: Workout details for the swim, bike, run, combination, and strength workouts are in Appendix A. If you don't have access to a gym, replace all strength workouts with resistance exercises, also found in Appendix A.

	THURSDAY	FRIDAY	SATURDAY	SUNDAY	
	Run #8 and optional strength #1	Swim #1 and optional bike #10	Bike #14	Run #1 and optional swim #1	
	Run #8 and optional strength #1	Swim #1 and optional bike #10	Bike #14	Run #2 and optional swim #1	
	Run #8 and optional strength #2	Swim #2 and optional bike #10	Bike #14	Run #3 and optional swim #1	
	Run #8 and optional strength #3	Swim #2 and optional bike #10	Bike #14	Run #4 and optional swim #1	
	Run #3 and optional strength #3	Swim #3 and optional bike #10	Bike #13	Run #4 and optional swim #1	
	Run #8 and optional strength #3	Swim #3 and optional bike #10	Bike #14	Run #5 and optional swim #1	
	Run #4	Swim #4 and optional bike #10	Run #5 and optional bike #13	Combination #1 and optional swim #1	
	Run #8	Swim #4 and optional bike #10	Run #6 and optional bike #10	Combination #2 and optional swim #1	
	Run #6	Swim #6 and optional bike #10	Bike #13 and optional swim #1	Swim #6 and combination #3	
	Run #7	Swim #6 and optional bike #10	Bike #13 and optional swim #1	Swim #6 and combination #4	
	Run #8	Swim #6 and optional bike #10	Bike #10 and optional swim #1	Swim #6 and combination #3	
	Swim #2	Bike #1	*YOUR FIRST TRIATHLON*	Day off	
	Run #1	Swim #2	Bike #1	*YOUR FIRST TRIATHLON*	

Sprint Plan

Table 9.4 Sprint Experienced Runner Plan

WEEKS TO TRI	MONDAY	TUESDAY	WEDNESDAY	
12	Optional strength #1 or day off	Swim #1 and optional run #9	Bike #1	
11	Optional strength #1 or day off	Swim #1 and optional run #9	Bike #2	
10	Optional strength #2 or day off	Swim #2 and optional run #9	Bike #1	
9 R&R	Optional strength #3 or day off	Swim #2 and optional run #9	Bike #5	
8	Optional strength #3 or day off	Swim #3 and optional run #8	Bike #1	
7	Optional strength #3 or day off	Swim #3 and optional run #9	Bike #7	
6 R&R	Optional strength #4 or day off	Swim #4 and optional run #8	Bike #7	
5	Optional strength #4 or day off	Swim #4 and optional run #9	Bike #9	
4	Optional strength #4 or day off	Swim #5 and optional run #8	Bike #8	
3 R&R	Optional strength #4 or day off	Swim #5 and optional run #8	Bike #8	
2	Optional strength #4 or day off	Swim #5 and optional run #9	Bike #9	
1 Saturday Race	Day off	Bike #3	Run #8	
1 Sunday Race	Day off	Swim #5	Bike #3	

Note: Workout details for the swim, bike, run, combination, and strength workouts are in Appendix A. If you don't have access to a gym, replace all strength workouts with resistance exercises, also found in Appendix A.

THURSDAY	FRIDAY	SATURDAY	SUNDAY
Run #8 and optional strength #1	Swim #1 and optional bike #1	Bike #2	Run #12 and optional swim #1
Run #8 and optional strength #1	Swim #1 and optional bike #1	Bike #3	Run #12 and optional swim #1
Run #8 and optional strength #2	Swim #2 and optional bike #3	Bike #4	Run #12 and optional swim #1
Run #8 and optional strength #3	Swim #2 and optional bike #3	Bike #9	Run #12 and optional swim #1
Run #9 and optional strength #3	Swim #3 and optional bike #1	Bike #9	Run #10 and optional swim #1
Run #11 and optional strength #3	Swim #3 and optional bike #3	Bike #10	Run #10 and optional swim #1
Run #11	Swim #4 and optional bike #3	Run #10	Combination #1 and optional swim #1
Run #11	Swim #4 and optional bike #2	Run #10	Combination #2 and optional swim #1
Run #11	Swim #6 and optional bike #3	Bike #9 and optional swim #1	Swim #6 and combination #3
Run #11	Swim #6 and optional bike #3	Bike #3 and optional swim #1	Swim #6 and combination #4
Run #8	Swim #6 and optional bike #1	Bike #1 and optional swim #1	Swim #6 and combination #3
Swim #2	Bike #1	*YOUR FIRST TRIATHLON*	Day off
Run #8	Swim #2	Bike #1	*YOUR FIRST TRIATHLON*

Sprint Plan

Table 9.5 Olympic Beginner Plan

WEEKS TO TRI	MONDAY	TUESDAY	WEDNESDAY	
12	Optional strength #1 or day off	Swim #9 and optional run #13	Bike #16	
11	Optional strength #1 or day off	Swim #9 and optional run #13	Bike #17	
10	Optional strength #2 or day off	Swim #10 and optional run #14	Bike #16	
9 R&R	Optional strength #3 or day off	Swim #10 and optional run #15	Bike #17	
8	Optional strength #3 or day off	Swim #11 and optional run #20	Bike #16	
7	Optional strength #3 or day off	Swim #11 and optional run #16	Bike #22	
6 R&R	Optional strength #4 or day off	Swim #12 and optional run #20	Bike #22	
5	Optional strength #4 or day off	Swim #12 and optional run #16	Bike #24	
4	Optional strength #4 or day off	Swim #13 and optional run #20	Bike #23	
3 R&R	Optional strength #4 or day off	Swim #13 and optional run #20	Bike #23	
2	Optional strength #4 or day off	Swim #13 and optional run #16	Bike #24	
1 Saturday Race	Day off	Bike #18	Run #13	
1 Sunday Race	Day off	Swim #10	Bike #18	

Note: Workout details for the swim, bike, run, combination, and strength workouts are in Appendix A. If you don't have access to a gym, replace all strength workouts with resistance exercises, also found in Appendix A.

THURSDAY	FRIDAY	SATURDAY	SUNDAY
Run #20 and optional strength #1	Swim #9 and optional bike #16	Bike #17	Run #13 and optional swim #9
Run #20 and optional strength #1	Swim #9 and optional bike #16	Bike #18	Run #14 and optional swim #9
Run #20 and optional strength #2	Swim #10 and optional bike #18	Bike #16	Run #15 and optional swim #9
Run #20 and optional strength #3	Swim #10 and optional bike #18	Bike #24	Run #16 and optional swim #9
Run #15 and optional strength #3	Swim #11 and optional bike #16	Bike #24	Run #16 and optional swim #9
Run #20 and optional strength #3	Swim #11 and optional bike #18	Bike #25	Run #17 and optional swim #9
Run #16	Swim #12 and optional bike #18	Run #17	Combination #5 and optional swim #9
Run #20	Swim #12 and optional bike #17	Run #18	Combination #6 and optional swim #9
Run #18	Swim #14 and optional bike #18	Bike #24 and optional swim #9	Swim #14 and combination #7
Run #19	Swim #14 and optional bike #18	Bike #18 and optional swim #9	Swim #14 and combination #8
Run #20	Swim #14 and optional bike #16	Bike #16 and optional swim #9	Swim #14 and combination #7
Swim #9	Bike #1	*YOUR FIRST TRIATHLON*	Day off
Run #13	Swim #9	Bike #1	*YOUR FIRST TRIATHLON*

Olympic Plan

Table 9.6 Olympic Experienced Swimmer Plan

WEEKS TO TRI	MONDAY	TUESDAY	WEDNESDAY	
12	Optional strength #1 or day off	Swim #7 and optional run #13	Bike #16	
11	Optional strength #1 or day off	Swim #7 and optional run #13	Bike #17	
10	Optional strength #2 or day off	Swim #7 and optional run #14	Bike #16	
9 R&R	Optional strength #3 or day off	Swim #7 and optional run #15	Bike #20	
8	Optional strength #3 or day off	Swim #7 and optional run #20	Bike #16	
7	Optional strength #3 or day off	Swim #7 and optional run #16	Bike #22	
6 R&R	Optional strength #4 or day off	Swim #7 and optional run #20	Bike #22	
5	Optional strength #4 or day off	Swim #7 and optional run #16	Bike #24	
4	Optional strength #4 or day off	Swim #7 and optional run #20	Bike #23	
3 R&R	Optional strength #4 or day off	Swim #7 and optional run #20	Bike #23	
2	Optional strength #4 or day off	Swim #7 and optional run #16	Bike #24	
1 Saturday Race	Day off	Bike #18	Run #13	
1 Sunday Race	Day off	Swim #13	Bike #18	

Note: Workout details for the swim, bike, run, combination, and strength workouts are in Appendix A. If you don't have access to a gym, replace all strength workouts with resistance exercises, also found in Appendix A.

THURSDAY	FRIDAY	SATURDAY	SUNDAY
Run #20 and optional strength #1	Swim #7 and optional bike #16	Bike #17	Run #13 and optional swim #8
Run #20 and optional strength #1	Swim #7 and optional bike #16	Bike #18	Run #14 and optional swim #8
Run #20 and optional strength #2	Swim #7 and optional bike #18	Bike #19	Run #15 and optional swim #8
Run #20 and optional strength #3	Swim #7 and optional bike #18	Bike #24	Run #16 and optional swim #8
Run #15 and optional strength #3	Swim #7 and optional bike #16	Bike #24	Run #16 and optional swim #8
Run #20 and optional strength #3	Swim #7 and optional bike #18	Bike #25	Run #17 and optional swim #8
Run #16	Swim #7 and optional bike #18	Run #20	Combination #5 and optional swim #8
Run #20	Swim #7 and optional bike #18	Run #18	Combination #6 and optional swim #8
Run #18	Swim #7 and optional bike #18	Bike #24 and optional swim #8	Swim #6 and combination #7
Run #19	Swim #7 and optional bike #18	Bike #18 and optional swim #8	Swim #6 and combination #8
Run #20	Swim #7 and optional bike #16	Bike #16 and optional swim #8	Swim #6 and combination #7
Swim #10	Bike #1	*YOUR FIRST TRIATHLON*	Day off
Run #13	Swim #4	Bike #1	*YOUR FIRST TRIATHLON*

Olympic Plan

Table 9.7 Olympic Experienced Cyclist Plan

WEEKS TO TRI	MONDAY	TUESDAY	WEDNESDAY	
12	Optional strength #1 or day off	Swim #9 and optional run #13	Bike #23	
11	Optional strength #1 or day off	Swim #9 and optional run #13	Bike #23	
10	Optional strength #2 or day off	Swim #10 and optional run #14	Bike #23	
9 R&R	Optional strength #3 or day off	Swim #10 and optional run #15	Bike #23	
8	Optional strength #3 or day off	Swim #11 and optional run #20	Bike #25	
7	Optional strength #3 or day off	Swim #11 and optional run #16	Bike #30	
6 R&R	Optional strength #4 or day off	Swim #12 and optional run #20	Bike #30	
5	Optional strength #4 or day off	Swim #12 and optional run #16	Bike #25	
4	Optional strength #4 or day off	Swim #13 and optional run #20	Bike #30	
3 R&R	Optional strength #4 or day off	Swim #13 and optional run #20	Bike #30	
2	Optional strength #4 or day off	Swim #13 and optional run #16	Bike #25	
1 Saturday Race	Day off	Bike #19	Run #13	
1 Sunday Race	Day off	Swim #10	Bike #19	

Note: Workout details for the swim, bike, run, combination, and strength workouts are in Appendix A. If you don't have access to a gym, replace all strength workouts with resistance exercises, also found in Appendix A.

	THURSDAY	FRIDAY	SATURDAY	SUNDAY
	Run #20 and optional strength #1	Swim #9 and optional bike #25	Bike #29	Run #13 and optional swim #9
	Run #20 and optional strength #1	Swim #9 and optional bike #25	Bike #29	Run #14 and optional swim #9
	Run #20 and optional strength #2	Swim #10 and optional bike #25	Bike #29	Run #15 and optional swim #9
	Run #20 and optional strength #3	Swim #10 and optional bike #25	Bike #29	Run #16 and optional swim #9
	Run #15 and optional strength #3	Swim #11 and optional bike #25	Bike #28	Run #16 and optional swim #9
	Run #20 and optional strength #3	Swim #11 and optional bike #25	Bike #29	Run #17 and optional swim #9
	Run #16	Swim #12 and optional bike #25	Run #17	Combination #5 and optional swim #9
	Run #20	Swim #12 and optional bike #25	Run #18	Combination #6 and optional swim #9
	Run #18	Swim #14 and optional bike #25	Bike #28 and optional swim #9	Swim #14 and combination #7
	Run #19	Swim #14 and optional bike #25	Bike #28 and optional swim #9	Swim #14 and combination #8
	Run #20	Swim #14 and optional bike #25	Bike #25 and optional swim #9	Swim #14 and combination #7
	Swim #9	Bike #16	*YOUR FIRST TRIATHLON*	Day off
	Run #13	Swim #9	Bike #16	*YOUR FIRST TRIATHLON*

Olympic Plan

Table 9.8 Olympic Experienced Runner Plan

WEEKS TO TRI	MONDAY	TUESDAY	WEDNESDAY	
12	Optional strength #1 or day off	Swim #9 and optional run #21	Bike #16	
11	Optional strength #1 or day off	Swim #9 and optional run #21	Bike #17	
10	Optional strength #2 or day off	Swim #10 and optional run #21	Bike #16	
9 R&R	Optional strength #3 or day off	Swim #10 and optional run #21	Bike #20	
8	Optional strength #3 or day off	Swim #11 and optional run #20	Bike #16	
7	Optional strength #3 or day off	Swim #11 and optional run #21	Bike #22	
6 R&R	Optional strength #4 or day off	Swim #12 and optional run #20	Bike #22	
5	Optional strength #4 or day off	Swim #12 and optional run #21	Bike #24	
4	Optional strength #4 or day off	Swim #13 and optional run #20	Bike #23	
3 R&R	Optional strength #4 or day off	Swim #13 and optional run #820	Bike #23	
2	Optional strength #4 or day off	Swim #13 and optional run #21	Bike #24	
1 Saturday Race	Day off	Bike #18	Run #20	
1 Sunday Race	Day off	Swim #10	Bike #18	

Note: Workout details for the swim, bike, run, combination, and strength workouts are in Appendix A. If you don't have access to a gym, replace all strength workouts with resistance exercises, also found in Appendix A.

Olympic Plan

THURSDAY	FRIDAY	SATURDAY	SUNDAY
Run #20 and optional strength #1	Swim #9 and optional bike #16	Bike #17	Run #24 and optional swim #9
Run #20 and optional strength #1	Swim #9 and optional bike #16	Bike #18	Run #24 and optional swim #9
Run #20 and optional strength #2	Swim #10 and optional bike #18	Bike #19	Run #24 and optional swim #9
Run #20 and optional strength #3	Swim #10 and optional bike #18	Bike #24	Run #24 and optional swim #9
Run #21 and optional strength #3	Swim #11 and optional bike #16	Bike #24	Run #22 and optional swim #9
Run #23 and optional strength #3	Swim #11 and optional bike #18	Bike #25	Run #22 and optional swim #9
Run #23	Swim #12 and optional bike #18	Run #22	Combination #5 and optional swim #9
Run #23	Swim #12 and optional bike #17	Run #22	Combination #6 and optional swim #9
Run #23	Swim #14 and optional bike #18	Bike #24 and optional swim #9	Swim #14 and combination #7
Run #23	Swim #14 and optional bike #18	Bike #18 and optional swim #9	Swim #14 and combination #8
Run #20	Swim #14 and optional bike #16	Bike #16 and optional swim #9	Swim #14 and combination #7
Swim #9	Bike #1	*YOUR FIRST TRIATHLON*	Day off
Run #20	Swim #9	Bike #1	*YOUR FIRST TRIATHLON*

Olympic Plan

Optional Workouts

In each plan, most weeks have two swim, two bike, and two run workouts scheduled. Beginning at six weeks to go until your first triathlon, combination (bike + run) workouts are included. There are also optional swim, bike, run, and strength workouts included for each week. These are workouts you may do if you have the time, but they aren't necessary if you just want to finish the triathlon. The experienced swimmer, cyclist, or runner may want to do the optional workout in his or her sport to maintain a higher level of fitness.

Combination Workouts

These training sessions, combining biking and running into one workout, are the key to doing well in triathlon once you've established a good level of base fitness. Over the course of several weeks they become mini-triathlons and prepare you for the challenge of completing two or more sports without rest.

Recovery and Rejuvenation (R&R) Weeks

Recovery and rejuvenation weeks are built into the plans at nine, six, and three weeks before your first triathlon. During these weeks consider cutting back even more if you are especially tired or feeling pressured to keep up with everything in your life. It is perfectly fine not to do the optional workouts or to leave out one or more of the primary workouts in order to rest more. These mini-breaks will allow you to physically rest and mentally rejuvenate. There will be no loss of fitness. In fact, after resting more than usual, you will probably feel as if you gained fitness.

Race Week

The last two weeks on each schedule are called "1 Week to Tri on Saturday" and "1 Week to Tri on Sunday." Follow only one of these weekly plans, depending on which day your first triathlon is to be held.

Should You Exercise with a Cold?

Training hard makes you a candidate for an upper respiratory infection. As the workload increases, so does the risk of catching a cold or the flu.

A few years ago a study of entrants in the Los Angeles Marathon (now called the Honda LA Marathon) found that those who ran more than 60 miles per week had twice as many illnesses as those running less than 20. Also, runners who completed the marathon were six times as likely to be ill the week following the race as those who registered but did not show up to run it.

What you do in the six hours following a hard workout or race is critical to your health. During this brief window of time, the immune system is depressed and less capable of fighting off disease. This is a good time to avoid people and public places. Wash your hands after any contact with others or with public facilities. Try to develop the habit of touching your face only with your nondominant hand and touching objects, such as doors and telephones, with your dominant hand. Take extra care of yourself for these six hours.

What should you do when, even after taking all these precautions, you feel a cold coming on—continue training as normal, reduce training, or completely rest? A "neck check" will help you decide. If you have above-the-neck symptoms, such as a runny nose or a scratchy throat, start your workout, but reduce the intensity and duration. You may begin to feel better after warming up, but if not, stop. If the symptoms are below the neck—such as a sore throat, chest cold, chills, coughing up matter, achy muscles, or a fever—don't even start. These are often symptoms of a really bad cold or even a virus. Exercising will make it worse.

Even after a flu bug departs, you're likely to experience a decrease in performance for some time. How long depends on the type and severity of the illness. One study found a 15 percent reduction in muscle strength that lasted up to a month following a virus. It may take three months to return to your

CONTINUED

CONTINUED

previous level of aerobic capacity after an especially bad case of the flu. During this time muscles may produce more lactic acid at lower levels of intensity than before the illness. You may also feel weak for some time.

Training with the flu will not bring improved fitness. Complete rest is needed. Let your body's energy reserves go into fighting the bug rather than trying to recover from workouts.

WHAT TO DO WHEN THINGS DON'T GO AS PLANNED

As I discussed previously, you're going to miss some workouts. An occasional missed workout will have no negative consequences for your first triathlon, but I must stress that repeatedly missing workouts, such as once or twice a week, will considerably reduce your fitness.

Although you can usually forget about the missed workout and continue on with your training plan as if nothing has happened, combination workouts should not be missed because they are very important to your preparation. If you can anticipate that you will miss one of these workouts, try rearranging your workouts for that week so that you can fit it in and leave out another one in the sport at which you are strongest. If you do the optional strength workouts, they should always be the first ones to omit.

On the other side of this when-things-don't-go-as-planned coin is the change an overly zealous athlete may make in the training plan to try to fit in more workouts or longer workouts. This is often a mistake that eventually causes greater problems down the road—usually in the form of burnout, illness, or injury. The key to success in your first triathlon is *not* how hard the training is, but rather how consistent it is. Doing more may seem alright at first, but it usually results in a setback sometime in the near future. You're better off sticking with the plan.

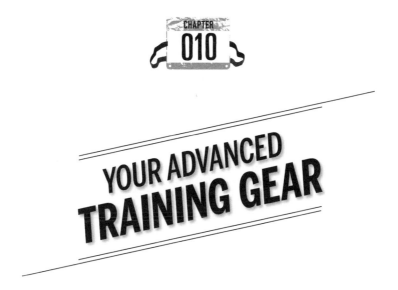

YOUR ADVANCED TRAINING GEAR

Chapters 5, 6, and 7 described the basic swim, bike, and run equipment you need for your first triathlon. This chapter takes a look at the more sophisticated training gear that is also used by many triathletes. While some of the equipment described here is becoming increasingly accessible, it still requires a considerable amount of dedicated use to master. These devices can help in some small ways to make you a better athlete; however, they are still just tools. You don't really *need* to use any of this stuff. The gear in this chapter has the potential to make your training more precise and could offer a slight boost to your fitness, but it's questionable whether a newcomer to the sport needs such precision. Your fitness will improve dramatically without any advanced technology.

Yet there are some people who simply like technology. I'm one of them. I've always enjoyed tinkering with gadgets that could measure and help me analyze what my body is experiencing when swimming, biking, and running. So if you're into technology, this chapter is for you. If not, skip this chapter and continue to keep training simple. Once you are thoroughly hooked on triathlon, you may start looking for ways to get a slight edge in fitness. That's when you'll come back to this chapter, because the equipment described here can make a difference.

There is more technology available for triathlon than for any other endurance sport. You can monitor heart rate, training zones, cycling power, pace, time, elevation, grade changes, and more if you have all the gear described here. Many triathletes do, and they spend nearly as much time analyzing data after workouts as they spend in training. Some have elaborate records of such training metrics going back years. A few have even created complex spreadsheets that allow them to easily enter and retrieve data. If you would like to collect such personal data but don't want the bother of building spreadsheets, go to the TrainingPeaks web site (www.TrainingPeaks.com), where easy upload and analysis functions are available for a small monthly subscription fee. You'll also discover lots of other features there to improve your training.

There are currently four gadgets to help track your swimming, cycling, and running—heart rate monitors, bicycle power meters, GPS devices, and accelerometers. Before buying any of these, do your research and then shop for the best deals. Following is a short discussion of these four pieces of equipment. Remember, they are not necessary, and by themselves they will not make you a better triathlete. As a matter of fact, most pro triathletes do not use high-tech stuff, preferring instead to simply swim, bike, and run based on how they feel.

HEART RATE MONITORS

When asked how hard you ran today you might say, "It was easy." This really doesn't tell the other person exactly what you did. So you could say, "On a scale of 1 to 5, with 5 being hardest, it was a 2." Rating of Perceived Exertion (RPE) is considerably more descriptive. You could also say, "I ran a 10-minute-per-mile pace on average." That's even more precise. You might even add, "My heart rate was about 130 beats per minute all the way." Of course, even though heart rate is a good way to express (and control) intensity, to have this continual feedback it is necessary to wear a heart rate monitor.

In 1978 a Finnish company, Polar Electro Oy, developed the first wireless, portable heart rate monitor and changed forever the way athletes in aerobic sports trained. A wireless heart rate monitor has two components. The chest strap has built-in sensors that pick up the electrical activity of the heart and then send the signal from a small radio transmitter to a receiver worn on the wrist like a watch. Besides displaying your heart rate, most receivers also include time of day and a stopwatch, and they have a memory function to record lap times and heart rate by zones.

Basic models that display only heart rate start at about $50. If you want all the bells and whistles plus the ability to download and manipulate data on your computer, expect to pay $400 or more. All types of heart rate monitors are available in triathlon, bike, running, and sporting goods stores, and through catalogs.

You don't have to use a heart rate monitor when training for your first triathlon, but it can help get the intensity right during workouts. Should you decide to buy one, there are two basic ways you can determine what your personal heart rate zones are. But before getting into that, let's address a couple of related matters. First of all, your heart rate during a workout is not likely to be the same as that of your training partner or spouse. There's a great deal of individuality when it comes to heart rate. So if yours is higher or lower than another person's even though you are working out together, do not be concerned. It doesn't mean either of you necessarily has a heart condition of some sort, or for that matter, any other health problem.

The second concern is that you shouldn't use 220 minus your age to estimate your maximum heart rate. This is as likely to be wrong as right. That was originally intended to be a way of estimating the average max heart rates of a large group of people. It works pretty well for that. But within any such group there will be great variation, with some having much higher or lower heart rates. Using the 220 formula is like throwing a dart at a dartboard covered with numbers ranging from 140 to 200.

So now let's get back to how to set up your zones. The first way to do this involves going to a lab or medical clinic to be tested. In fact, this is a good idea even if you don't have a heart rate monitor. Not only will a "stress test" administered by a professional give you heart rate data, but it will also confirm that your heart is healthy and ready for training. This is something triathletes should do periodically whether they use a heart rate monitor or not. Such a test generally costs $150 or more.

What you want to find out from such testing, other than fitness status, is your lactate threshold (sometimes called "anaerobic threshold") heart rate. Make sure the test technician knows what heart rate information you are after and why. You're likely to test in only one sport—bike or run—but you can estimate the one not tested. If you ran on a treadmill, subtract eight beats per minute from the lactate threshold heart rate (LTHR) to estimate bike LTHR. If the test was done on a bike ergometer, add eight beats per minute to estimate run LTHR.

The second way to determine your heart rate zones is to do what's called a "field test." This is a workout you do on your own while in the real world, not in a lab, and of course it's free. See the "How to Find Your Heart Rate Zones" sidebar for an explanation of how to do this. If you did the lab test, also use this sidebar to determine your personal zones.

Although it's possible to use a heart rate monitor while swimming, don't do so unless you are an experienced swimmer. Remember that your purpose in the pool for now is to develop good swim technique, not fitness. The latter will come as a result of working on your skills. But if you are an experienced swimmer, you can subtract eight beats per minute from your bike LTHR to estimate swim LTHR and then set up zones (see the "How to Find Your Heart Rate Zones" sidebar).

POWER METERS

Power meters are fairly recent additions to the triathlete's cycling equipment arsenal, having been around since only the early 1990s. Whereas a heart rate monitor tells you how hard your body is working (input), a

How to Find Your Heart Rate Zones

When using a heart rate monitor during exercise, you need a standard to which your target heart rate can be compared. I like to use lactate threshold heart rate (LTHR) for this marker.

Running Field Test: To find yours for running, go to a track, and after warming up for 10 minutes, start running slowly around it. Every half lap (200 meters), increase your speed just a little (about 2 to 4 seconds faster per 200), paying close attention to your breathing and effort. Continue this speed increase until you first notice the onset of rapid and deep breathing while experiencing a feeling of hard effort (RPE 4), look at your heart rate monitor. Your heart rate at this time will be pretty close to your LTHR.

Cycling Field Test: A similar method can be used to find your LTHR for the bike. On a long, gradual hill or a stretch of flat road without stop signs, start riding easily and slightly increase the effort every 30 seconds. When you first start to breathe rapidly and deeply (RPE 4), look at your heart rate monitor. The number is close to your LTHR.

Another way of gauging LTHR during a run or a bike workout that gradually becomes harder is to simply use RPE alone to gauge how hard you are running or biking on a scale of 1 to 5, with 5 being the hardest. Your LTHR is about 4 on this scale.

Once you know your LTHR for a sport, you can determine your five heart rate training zones. Here's how:

Zone 1. This is the easiest zone. You will spend a lot of time in the first zone warming up, on very easy days, and cooling down. If you are new to running, zone 1 will probably be walking. On the bike, zone 1 is like walking on your bike—very easy.

My run zone 1 is less than _____ beats per minute (subtract 24 bpm from run LTHR)

My bike zone 1 is less than _____ beats per minute (subtract 31 bpm from bike LTHR)

CONTINUED

CONTINUED

Zone 2. This is the aerobic training zone, the one you will use to improve your basic endurance and aerobic fitness. For the running newbie, zone 2 is slow jogging. For biking you're just starting to push the pedals a bit.

My run zone 2 is _____ – _____ (15–23 bpm below run LTHR)

My bike zone 2 is _____ – _____ (17–30 bpm below bike LTHR)

Zone 3. Use this zone occasionally in workouts to improve race pace. When running or biking, this is when you first start to feel uncomfortable, but you know you could keep going for a long time.

My run zone 3 is _____ – _____ (7–14 bpm below run LTHR)

My bike zone 3 is _____ – _____ (10–16 bpm below bike LTHR)

Zone 4. This is a hard effort, which you will not use at the beginning. But someday, after you become an experienced triathlete, you will use this zone, especially when preparing for sprint- and Olympic-distance races.

My run zone 4 is _____ – _____ (1–6 bpm below run LTHR)

My bike zone 4 is _____ – _____ (1–9 bpm below bike LTHR)

Zone 5. Above LTHR is zone 5—redline effort. Do not use this zone at all, as the risk of injury is higher and recovery takes much longer. Even after you gain experience in the sport there is little need to train this intensely.

My run zone 5 is above _____ beats per minute (run LTHR)

My bike zone 5 is above _____ beats per minute (bike LTHR)

power meter tells you what you are accomplishing (output measured in watts). You might ask why you couldn't simply look at the speedometer on your handlebar computer to know what your output is. The problem with speed on a bike is that it is tremendously affected by outside influences such as wind and hills. If, for example, you told me that you completed a bike ride at an average speed of 18 mph, I wouldn't know what that meant. If it was all downhill with a tailwind, that would have been a pretty low output. The same speed done uphill or into a strong headwind, however, could have been quite an accomplishment. The same problem applies whether you are drafting another bike rider or riding by yourself. Speed is simply not a good measuring tool of output on the bike.

What power tells us is how much work you did per unit of time. Wind, hills, and drafting have no effect on it. If you told me you completed a ride at an average of 180 watts I would know exactly what that meant regardless of any other outside factors such as hills and wind.

As of this writing, five types of power meters are available. The manufacturers are PowerTap (www.cycle-ops.com), Quarq (www.quarq.com), and SRM (www.srm.de). In a separate category of power meters are devices made by iBike (www.ibikesports.com) and Polar (www.polarusa .com). These last two don't actually measure power directly as the first three products do, but rather estimate it using complex algorithms based on other available data. They aren't quite as accurate, but they are reliable. That makes these two far less costly than the first three.

The least expensive power meter is the iBike ($400) and the most expensive is the SRM ($2,400). As these prices imply, there is a significant difference between products. Because this is a rapidly changing market, you should consult the manufacturer web sites for more information.

GPS DEVICES

Using the government's Global Positioning System (GPS) satellites, these wristwatch-type devices allow you not only to keep track of where you are on the planet but also to compute your real-time pace or speed, distance traveled, elevation, and hill gradients. They are especially helpful to use while running, since without such a device you have no idea what your pace is other than by guessing or running on a track while constantly translating lap splits into pace. A GPS device can also be used on your bike in place of the handlebar computer and can give you all the same information and more—time, current speed, average speed, distance, elevation, and hill grade. Some tell you heart rate, too. And they don't care if you are on a winding trail or a major thoroughfare, in the desert or a city park, on a mountain or by the seashore. So long as you can see the sky, it's working and telling you what you're accomplishing (or not accomplishing).

Prices for GPS watches start at about $250. Companies that make endurance sport GPS devices as of this writing are Garmin (www.garmin .com), Polar (www.polarusa.com), and Timex (www.timex.com). There are also apps available for smartphones that turn them into GPS training gear. Again, check with manufacturers for the most current information.

ACCELEROMETERS

Watches for runners have come a long way since my first one back in 1979. All it did was tell time and provide a stopwatch. Accelerometers are the latest cool addition to the high-tech runner's arsenal. Like a GPS device, it measures speed and distance. It doesn't offer altitude or hill gradient information, however. The working end of the accelerometer is usually a small "pod" that attaches to your shoelaces. This is a highly precise instrument that measures acceleration and deceleration of the foot hundreds of times per second. It's far more precise than a pedometer and doesn't require entering a standard stride length. The foot pod transmits data to a wristwatch that converts it to speed and distance. The wristwatch also provides heart rate along with the standard timing data. Unlike a GPS, an accelerometer does not need to "see" the sky to work effectively. So you can run in a forest or among skyscrapers without losing data. An accelerometer is typically less expensive than a GPS. They can be found for less than $200.

Companies making accelerometers for runners are Nike (www.nike .com), Polar (www.polarusa.com), Suunto (www.suunto.com), Tech4o (www.tech4o.com), and Timex (www.timex.com).

The latest use of accelerometers is for pool swimming. Finis, a leader in the field of swim equipment and clothing, has developed a device that keeps track of your distance (meters/yards/laps), stroke count, stroke rate, distance per stroke, and calories burned. It's called the Swimsense (www.finisinc.com/equipment/electronics/swimsense.html). All these data are captured in a small wristwatch and can be downloaded to your computer after the swim. As of this writing it retails for about $200.

BACK TO THE FUTURE

Manufacturers are well on their way to combining the abilities of these devices into one product that can do it all. With data readouts wirelessly transmitted to sunglasses, athletes will be like fighter pilots with "heads-up" displays, never having to take their eyes off where they are going. As of this writing, one company has just released such a product (www.4iiii .com).

Here's a far-out thought. Really serious athletes may eventually have a tiny chip medically embedded to monitor heart rate, blood sugar, blood sodium, body acidity, velocity, power, elevation, distance, and gradient, all while predicting performance outcome. All the data would be transmitted to a heads-up display or to an earpiece and might even be presented as a single number called "Rating of Perceived Exertion." We'd then be right back where we started, only in a high-tech way. That's fun stuff for techies to ponder.

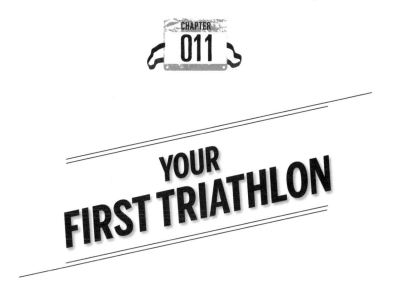

YOUR FIRST TRIATHLON

Triathlon's active lifestyle is fun and rewarding, but the races can be a bit intimidating, perhaps even downright scary. And the closer you get to race day, the scarier it can become. The mere thought of the race may cause your heart to beat a little faster and give you an uneasy feeling. Why is this? Why is it you can swim, bike, and run with friends or alone and never feel anything but joy, yet become anxious, nervous, and apprehensive when going to or even thinking about a triathlon? Fear of the unknown, or a fear of failure, is very common.

Self-confidence is the best way to control your fear, even if it doesn't completely disappear. Remind yourself that you're doing everything you can to get in shape and that you're making good progress. Also, the more you know about what to expect at the race, the less intimidating race day becomes. I will give you clear expectations for both the race and the days and hours leading up to it.

You're likely to still be a bit edgy as you count down to your first triathlon. All triathletes experience this feeling, even those who have been doing it for years. Indeed, this is *the* test. It's what you've been preparing to do for many, many weeks. No one wants to perform poorly, and you won't if your race-day attitude is right. You need to go to the start line with a calm demeanor, confident that you have done the work and that you're ready to go. Let's race!

RACE WEEK

During the week of the race you may feel a bit strange because you'll be cutting back on exercise quite a bit to allow for rest. Although the extra time you have this week will feel good, it can also make you a little uneasy and even anxious. You'll probably feel you aren't doing enough and that your hard-earned fitness is fading away. But rest assured that it isn't. In fact, you are gaining race readiness by backing off this week. It's only during periods of low activity that the body gets rested up enough to race well. I've seen many triathletes—including very experienced ones who should know better—ruin their chances for good races by doing too much the week of their triathlons. Take it easy this week and fight off the self-doubt that tells you to do more. You'll do best by resting.

If you're following a training plan in Chapter 9, you'll find that your daily exercise has been reduced considerably. It's best to keep the rest of your week, as much as possible, like normal until the day before the race. This includes meals, sleep, work, and other activities.

THE DAY BEFORE

If the race is in your hometown or close by, the day before won't be too unusual. You'll sleep in your own bed and eat at home. That can be quite an advantage in keeping anxiety at bay. If you have to travel to the race, this is the day most people do it, although it's not necessarily the best from a racing perspective. Arriving two days before would be better because it keeps stress levels lower. But you may be unable to fit that around your job and other responsibilities.

Today's Workout

This morning do a short workout. The training plan suggested in Chapter 9 calls for a bike ride to give you one last chance to make sure everything is working. Should there be some little mechanical problem, you've still got time to get it to a bike shop. Even if everything is in good order after the ride, it's wise to check all the bolts to make sure they are snug. Don't overtighten them; you may break or strip a bolt. Just ensure that nothing is loose.

A few triathlons ask that you check in your bike the day before the race. Be sure to plan a morning ride well before the check-in time if this is a requirement of your triathlon.

Packet Pickup

More than likely you will have to pick up your race packet today. Bigger races often tie this in with an expo where vendors display their wares. It can be fun to see what is available for triathletes. Just be careful not to spend too much time on your legs; you want to rest them as much as possible today.

The packet will probably contain your race number or numbers, a course map with directions, comments on the rules of racing a triathlon (be sure to read this), a diagram of the transition area, start times by age group or ability, and sponsor information. The race number usually has a perforated portion with your name, age, and perhaps other identification. Check this to make sure it's correct before leaving the expo area.

You may also find a timing chip in the packet. This is a small electronic device that fastens to your ankle and electronically identifies you. It is used to keep track of where you are on the course and your "splits"—the times of the individual swim, bike, and run legs of the race. Be sure to follow the instructions about how to wear your race chip.

Know the Course

Even if you are familiar with the racecourse, today is a good time to drive it again to see if anything has changed. If you are doing a destination race and you have never seen the course, this is imperative. Race directors often paint arrows on the road at all the turns, so with a course map and by watching for the arrows you should be able to find your way easily. Even though there are likely to be lots of other racers and course marshals to direct you on race day, it's your responsibility to know the route. Pay close attention to hills and dangerous intersections. Police should be on hand to control traffic for the race, but it's still a good idea to know what to expect.

Race Briefing

At this meeting, usually held the day before the triathlon, the race organizers explain what will happen on race day, including details about any changes to the course, how the transition area is set up, and any other last-minute updates. You can also expect to hear a lot of questions from nervous athletes. If there is such a meeting for entrants, you should attend even if it is not required.

Before you leave home, check the race information (online or in a packet mailed to you) to learn when and where the race briefing will be held. Arrive well in advance to allow time to get to the meeting without feeling rushed. You will want to keep everything you do today as relaxed as possible.

Eating and Drinking

You may need to change your diet a bit today to help prevent an upset stomach at the race. Breakfast can be your normal fare, but for the remainder of the day it may be best to avoid fibrous foods and to eat lighter than usual. Soft foods (such as a baked potato) and soup or other liquid food sources are good choices for the night before your first triathlon.

Endurance athletes tend to go overboard drinking fluids the day before a hot race. You're not a camel, so you won't be able to store huge amounts of fluid. You'll simply pee more and are likely to dilute your electrolytes by drinking copious amounts. As always, just drink enough to quench your thirst.

Some triathlons offer a carbo-loading or pasta party the night before the race. This can be a fun experience, and you'll meet lots of other tri-athletes there. Again, expect almost everyone to be nervous and uptight. Don't let their concerns and agitation get to you. Remain calm and re-laxed even if others around you are frazzled.

Race Gear Preparation

The evening before your race is a good time to get all the stuff you'll need on race day organized and ready to go. Start by laying out all your swim gear together. Make a second grouping of your bike gear minus the bike. Then put the run equipment together. Double-check your lists to make sure you have everything (see Appendix B).

Fasten your race number to your shirt or race belt and put it on to en-sure it complies with the race director's instructions about how to wear it. They usually require a number on your back (and on the bike) during the bike portion and on your front during the run. If this is the case and they gave you only one number to wear on your body, an elastic race belt is the answer.

If there is only one transition area for your race, put all your gear, along with your timing chip, in a bag or a backpack to be carried to the race the next morning. But leave your swimsuit out, because you will wear it to the race. If there are two transition areas (it's best not to do such a race for your first triathlon), pack two separate bags, making dou-ble sure you have only swim and bike gear in one and run stuff in the other.

Check the weather forecast for your race. That will help you decide what other clothes to take with you, such as sweats, arm covers, gloves, a raincoat, an umbrella, or various other warm-, cold-, or wet-weather gear. In general, I recommend taking more clothes than you think are necessary. I've seen race-day weather unexpectedly turn nasty, catching athletes by surprise. The worst thing that could happen if you take extra clothes is that you'd have to carry them in and out of the transition area on race day. Load the extra clothes into a separate backpack, which may wind up staying in the trunk of the car tomorrow. But at least you know you have them just in case.

Keep Your Mind off the Race

If you traveled to the race early and have a lot of time to kill today, it's best to stay away from other entrants so you can keep your mind off the race. Also, stay off your legs once you've done your morning workout (more on this shortly). Read a book, watch television, or go to a movie. If you're in a city you haven't visited before, another fun and relaxing option is to sign up for a bus tour of the area. The hotel can help you find such a service.

Sleep

Go to bed tonight at about your normal time or slightly earlier. If you're in a strange bed and a different time zone, especially if you traveled east, this may be a bit difficult. To help you get sleepy, turn the lights down low an hour or so before bedtime, read a book, or watch TV. Now is not the time to party with other triathletes.

RACE MORNING

The big day is finally here—the culmination of weeks of focused preparation. You're nervous, but that's normal. If you weren't a bit anxious I would be concerned. I like to see the athletes I coach just a bit on edge on race day. That means they'll be in the right frame of mind and race well.

Avoid thinking about what your finishing time will be or how you will place in your age group. Stop worrying about finishing last—you won't! Avoid undue pressure to perform today. With the possible exception of your mother, no one expects you to win the race. You're out there to have fun and just finish. So relax and enjoy the experience. There's nothing else like it in the world of sport.

Sleeping, Eating, and Other Problems

You may not have slept much, if at all, the night before. That's pretty common for triathletes at all levels. Don't let it concern you. If you slept satisfactorily two nights before, your race will still go well. Get up an hour or so before you have to drive to the race venue but no less than three hours before your start time. That will allow you to wake up, perhaps drink a cup of coffee, eat a light breakfast, get dressed, and use the bathroom.

If you are in from out-of-town it's best to pack what you'll need for your race-day breakfast or purchase food at a grocery store the day before. The food you eat today should be easy to digest, as your stomach is likely to be squeamish. Eat only foods you have eaten before workouts. Generally, it's not a good idea to do anything today that you haven't tried before in training.

Some foods that may go down easily for you today are oatmeal, unsweetened applesauce, banana, sports food supplements (such as GatorPro), liquid meals in a bottle (such as Ensure), and energy bars with water. Although this may sound weird, baby food is also easy to digest and is used by some athletes on race day. Triathletes use a wide variety of foods before races; hopefully you have experimented with various foods before some of your workouts and know what works best for you.

Assuming you're awake and up about three hours before your race start time, consume about 200–400 calories, depending on your size, appetite, and how nervous you feel. For example, a banana is 100–140 calories depending on size, 1 cup of oatmeal is about 190 calories, and 1 cup of unsweetened applesauce is approximately 100 calories. Don't skip breakfast today—even a little bit of food will prove helpful. Try to be done with your breakfast no less than two hours before the race start.

Before leaving your room try to use the bathroom. Drinking hot coffee, tea, or even warm water as soon as you get up may help. This will be a lot more comfortable in your home or hotel than in a portable toilet at the race.

What to Wear

On the morning of the race, put on what you will wear for the swim portion of the triathlon. This may be a swimsuit or a one- or two-piece triathlon suit. You may want to wear some shorts and a T-shirt or a sweat suit
over this. Check one last time to make sure you have your race numbers,
timing chip, and swim, bike, and run gear before heading out the door.

Arrive Early

Plan to arrive at the race venue 60–90 minutes before your start time.
For some big races, 60 minutes may be cutting it close because of having
to park and then walk to the transition area. You don't want to feel hur-
ried and hassled. Allow enough time so that you can move at a leisurely
pace and remain cool and calm. There are also a few things that must be
done for race check-in, and these can take time.

Race Check-In

Triathlon check-in on race day can take 10–20 minutes. One of the first
things you'll do is go through "body marking." This is usually right at the
entrance to the transition area. A volunteer will ask to see your race number and then will use a marker to write the number on your arm and leg.
Your age or age-group code will also be written on your leg, usually on
the calf. The race numbers identify you during the swim. The age mark
lets your fellow triathletes know what age group you are in during the
race.

If your bike wasn't checked in yesterday, a volunteer may need to do a
safety check to make sure the handlebars are tight and the brakes work.
Your helmet may also be checked to ensure that it complies with U.S.
Consumer Product Safety Commission (CPSC) or Snell safety standards
for bicycle helmets (there should be a sticker inside that indicates this).

You're now ready to go into the transition area and rack your bike.
The next order of business is to check that your tires are pumped up
appropriately and then to set up your personal transition space. If you

don't have a pump, borrow one from another racer or a race official. Bring your tire pressure up to about the level indicated on the sidewall of the tires. If it looks as if it might rain or the pavement is wet, keep the tire pressure a little low. It will be safer cornering that way.

The Transition Area

One of the things that makes triathlon such a unique sport is that the outcome is determined, in part, by how fast you can change from one sport to the next. This is called "transition" and is done in a special, usually fenced-in, area for athletes only.

Following the swim you will hustle to the transition area to prepare for the bike portion of the race. This is called "transition #1" or "T1." After the bike ride you will come back to the transition area again and change equipment to start the run. This is "T2." Time spent in the transition area changing shoes, putting your helmet on or taking it off, and doing everything else necessary to get out on the course again counts as a part of your total race time. The clock doesn't stop until you cross the finish line. For your first triathlon, don't be concerned about your time. But you do want your transitions to be smooth and efficient.

Since you are not allowed to have anyone help you, it's wise to organize your personal transition space and to rehearse your transitions several times in the final weeks before the race. The best time to rehearse T2 is when you do the combination or "brick" workouts described in Appendix A. T1 is a bit easier to do than T2.

T1 and T2 are usually in the same area, but in a few races there may be two entirely different transition sites. This is rare for sprint- and Olympic-distance races but could be the case for yours. Be sure to find out well in advance. When the transitions are in different locations, often separated by a few miles, organizing them is more difficult and even more critical. It's easy to make a setup mistake. If, for example, your running shoes are placed at T1 or your helmet is at T2, you won't be able to continue and will be listed by the race director as a "DNF"—did not finish.

YOUR TRANSITION STALL

The race director often designates your personal transition stall. If this is the case, you will set up your transition gear in that small, assigned space. If you are free to set up your stall wherever you want in the transition

Transition Checklist

This checklist is by transition area and lists all the equipment you must have or may want:

Transition #1 (Swim-to-Bike)	Required	Optional
Bike	✔	
Helmet	✔	
Race number (may be on bike and/or a belt or pinned to shirt)	✔	
T-shirt or singlet	✔	
Bike shoes (you can bike in running shoes, and many do for sprint triathlons)		✔
Socks (many triathletes race without them, but practice this first)		✔
Water bottle with sports drink (good idea)		✔
Sunglasses		✔
Cold weather gear (gloves, jacket, arm covers, etc.)		✔
Heart rate monitor chest strap		✔
Towel (beneficial)		✔
Transition #2 (Bike-to-Run)		
Running shoes (if you bike in them you're set)	✔	
Race number (may already be on shirt or belt)	✔	
Sunglasses (may already be on from bike ride)		✔
Hat		✔

Note: Also refer to Appendix B on page 221.

area, it is usually a good idea to locate it near the T1 exit—the place where you leave transition to head out on the bike course. This is especially important if you will be wearing bike shoes instead of running shoes in the bike segment. In this location you can put your bike shoes on and then walk or run slowly with your bike to the exit where you can mount it, with minimal time spent jogging in clumsy bike shoes.

At the end of your bike ride, when you are approaching the transition—about 100 yards or so before you get there—slow down by coasting. If you have clipless pedals, you can save some time if you unfasten your shoes and slip your feet out. Completely remove one first and then the other. Put your feet on the top of the shoes to finish pedaling easily to T2. Stop the bike and step off when instructed to do so. This will be just before the entrance to T2. Then you can run the bike to your stall barefoot with your shoes hanging from the pedals. This can be tricky, so be sure to practice several times before race day. This second run through the transition area with your bike will be longer but easier without clunky bike shoes on your feet. If you bike in running shoes, none of this is necessary, and you can set up your stall wherever it's convenient.

TRANSITION SETUP

Now let's take a look at how to organize your equipment at your personal transition stall. The transition area will generally have a simple bike rack made from pipes that looks like a big sawhorse or barricade. There are two ways you can put your bike on it. You can place the brake levers over the top of the rack so that it hangs from the handlebars with the front wheel off the ground, or you can place the nose of the saddle over the top of the rack so that the rear wheel is suspended. Either way is common, but the second may be necessary if you have some types of aerobars, or if you're riding a mountain bike or other bike with flat or straight handlebars. The race director may even specify how it is to be racked. If so, this will be in the instructions in your race packet or may be described at the pre-race meeting. Look around to see how others are racking their bikes.

Mount your water bottle—filled with the sports drink of your choice and ready to go—on your bike on race morning. You'll only need one such bottle on the bike for a sprint- or Olympic-distance race. On the run there will be aid stations, so you won't need to carry any bottles then.

Once your bike is racked, set up your transition stall. Start by spreading a bath towel on the ground on the opposite side of the bike from the chain. On this towel place your bike shoes (if you will be using these). Put them on the end of the towel farthest from the rack with the straps unfastened and as open as you can get them. If using running shoes instead, place them in the same manner.

On top of your shoes place your socks (if you will be using them). Most triathletes don't because it is difficult to put socks on wet feet. During your practices, try biking and running a few times without socks to see how you do. If you get hotspots or blisters on your feet, it's best to take a few seconds to put on socks in the transition. In this case find the socks that go on the easiest with damp feet. Try this a few times before race day.

Next, place your running shoes (if you don't ride in them) on the opposite end of the towel with the toes pointing away from you so you can easily slip into them. The laces should be loose and the tongue open wide for quick entry. This is where elastic laces or "lace locks" come in handy, as tying shoes in transition can be clumsy. These lacing systems are inexpensive and can be purchased in most running and triathlon stores. They are worth the small cost. Trying to tie laces while breathing hard and in a hurry usually means the laces will soon come untied.

Place your running cap upside down on top of your running shoes so you can quickly slap it on before putting on your shoes.

If you are using aerobars, lay your helmet upside down on the handlebars with the chin strap unclasped and the straps spread wide. The front of the helmet should point toward your saddle. If you are not using aerobars, lay your helmet upside down on top of your hat and running shoes. In either case, place your sunglasses inside your helmet opened up, with the lenses down.

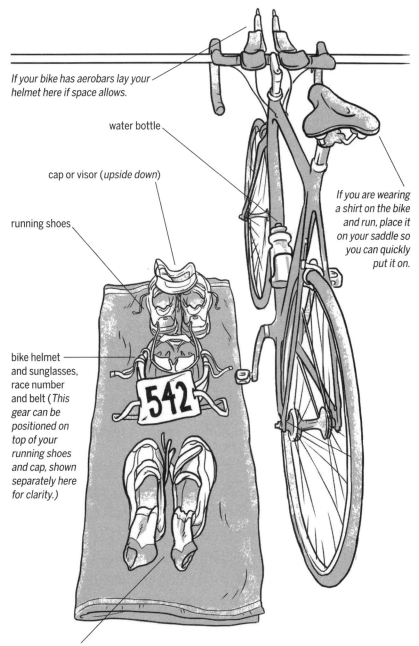

If your bike has aerobars lay your helmet here if space allows.

water bottle

cap or visor (*upside down*)

running shoes

If you are wearing a shirt on the bike and run, place it on your saddle so you can quickly put it on.

bike helmet and sunglasses, race number and belt (*This gear can be positioned on top of your running shoes and cap, shown separately here for clarity.*)

542

bike shoes and socks (*If you are using running shoes for the bike leg, they will be placed here.*)

Lay the shirt you will wear on the bike and the run on your saddle in such a way that you can slip it on. Make sure you find one that goes on easily when you are wet. Practice this several times in the last couple of weeks before the race.

It's not necessary, and may prove to be somewhat of a distraction, but if you're used to biking and running while watching your heart rate, you may want to wear your heart rate monitor in the triathlon; most triathletes do. If you want to, open the chest strap clasp and lay it on top of your shirt.

Most races require you to have a race number both on your bike and on your body throughout the bike and the run. If there is a number to be placed on your bike, the race instructions will explain where it is to be mounted. If the race gives you two identical numbers to be worn on your body throughout the bike and run portions, you can pin these to your shirt's front and back the night before. If they give you only one number, which is common, get a cheap elastic race belt with an easy-to-use clasp and use a safety pin to secure the number to the middle portion of it that would normally be on your backside when the belt is worn. Start the bike leg of the race with the belt slid around so that the number is on your back where race officials can easily see it. Then when you start the run, you can simply slide the belt around your waist so that the buckle is on the back and the number is on the front, where race officials can once again easily see it as you're approaching the finish line. Again, be sure to try this belt several times when rehearsing T1 and T2.

If you wear a race number belt during the race, lay it on top of your sunglasses and helmet with the buckle unclasped.

The setup I've described here may sound overly structured, but I can tell you from experience that if you do it this way your race will be much smoother, as you'll know where everything is and there will be no fumbling. There is more panic and chaos during transition than at any other time in a triathlon. Most of this comes from those who are sloppy and unprepared. A bit of structure and some rehearsal will make the day much more fun for you.

Warm-Up

For your first triathlon you won't need much of a warm-up, if any at all. If this is a pool swim, all lanes will probably be in use anyway, making it impossible to get a swim warm-up. If it is a lake or ocean swim it's okay to get in a short warm-up if the race director allows it. Treat the race like a workout and start out slowly. Race directors seldom allow bikes out of the transition area before the race starts, and running really doesn't do much to prepare you for a swim. Since your purpose today is to enjoy and to learn from the experience of finishing your first triathlon, starting the race slowly to get warmed up is not a problem. You'll simply do better beginning this way rather than trying to be a rocket ship from the start.

RACE START

Most triathlons start in waves—small groups of athletes separated by a few minutes. In open-water swims the groups are usually determined by age. In pool swims, predicted swim finish times are often used, since there will be two or more people in a lane and it makes things smoother if they are of similar ability. For pool swims your predicted swim time is generally asked for on the entry form. This should be based on times you get when practicing, especially the timed 400s called for every few weeks in the training plan in Chapter 9.

The race instructions should tell you when to report to the pool or shoreline. When that time arrives, take your goggles with you to the swim check-in. You may also be required to wear the swim cap provided in your race packet.

The Swim

For a pool swim you will start in the water, holding on to the wall. If there are just two of you in a lane, you will probably be told to divide the lane in half, with each of you staying to your own side near the lane rope. If there are three or more in the lane, you'll swim a counterclockwise, circular pattern, always staying to the right side of the lane. Start slowly but steadily.

Be aware of the other swimmers in your lane if there are three in a lane. You're not trying to beat them, but you also don't want to hinder them. There is a certain etiquette that must be followed. The most important has to do with passing. If the swimmer behind touches your feet then, the next time you come to the wall, stay to the right, pause holding on to the wall, and allow him or her to pass. Then continue swimming.

In an open-water swim you may start either in the water or on the beach, running into the water at the start command. In either case, since this is your first triathlon, it's best to start in the back row and off to one side. Don't go to the middle of the front row. Open-water swim starts are notorious for how rough they are, especially in the front middle. Experienced triathletes describe this as like being in a washing machine with flying hands and elbows and kicking feet. It's not a fun place to be. Avoid it.

Don't be in a hurry during the swim. Do it just as you've done in swim practice—slow and steady. Stop whenever you feel like it. There is no penalty for stopping at any time in the race regardless of which leg of the event it is. In an open-water swim there will be boats, kayaks, or surfboards scattered along the course. Find one of these and hang on to it for a little while if you feel the need. You won't be the only one.

If it is a pool swim, a race official on deck will count your laps and tell you when it's time to stop. In an open-water swim you will follow buoys that mark the course; pause and look around occasionally to make sure you are on course. Coming to the end of your swim, you may find it a bit difficult to stand up and run to T1. You may be a bit wobbly and not have your land legs for a few seconds. So climb out of the pool, lake, or ocean and cautiously stand up, taking a moment to regain your balance.

Transition #1

Walk or jog slowly from the water to your transition stall. With T1 laid out as described earlier in this chapter, making the switch from swim to bike should be a piece of cake. Pull on your socks (if applicable), slip into your shoes, put on your shirt and/or race number belt (with the number on your back), don your sunglasses, and plop on your helmet and buckle it. Then grab your bike off the rack and walk it to the bike exit. Be very careful if you have bike shoes on because they are rather clumsy to walk in. Once you're out of T1, a race official will tell you when you can mount your bike and start riding.

The Bike

Ride your bike just as you have done in practice dozens of times. Don't get into a head-to-head race with other triathletes. You're out here to have fun and finish the race; you're not here to beat someone or to see how fast you can go. Save that for your second triathlon. Look around and enjoy the experience today. Shout words of encouragement to other triathletes.

There are a couple of rules you need to be aware of, which the race director probably discussed in the pre-race meeting yesterday. The first has to do with "drafting," which isn't allowed in your triathlon. Drafting is following closely behind another rider, which makes the going pretty easy and is considered an unfair advantage in a triathlon. Be sure to read about this in the race instructions and listen closely when the race director talks about it in the pre-race meeting. You may be penalized or disqualified for drafting.

The other rule has to do with "blocking." This means riding to the left side of the bike course, forcing others to pass you on the right side. In effect they are being blocked from passing you on the left side. The best way to avoid a receiving penalty or being disqualified for blocking is to stay near the right curb except when passing.

Be sure to use your bottle of sports drink on the bike. For the sprint and Olympic race distances you won't need anything more. A couple of big sips every few minutes will keep you fueled all the way through the bike.

As you get close to the end of the bike course, sit up, slow down, and watch for course officials notifying you to get off your bike. About 100 yards or so before the finish, if you are wearing bike shoes, coast while you unfasten the straps and slip your feet out. Watch where you are going, and place your feet on top of the shoes by feel. Continue pedaling to the bike dismount area at the T2 entrance.

Transition #2

Approach T2 by gradually slowing down. Don't try to make up time or work hard to pass others in the last 100 yards. This can be a dangerous area if a lot of triathletes are finishing at the same time. Some will be going too fast, and others will be going so slow that they are wobbly and weave all over the road. Just ride a straight line and focus on what's happening ahead.

When an official tells you to dismount, come to a complete stop and get off your bike, leaving your bike shoes attached to the pedals. Then jog or walk with your bike to your transition stall. Rack your bike the same way it was when you came to T1. Step onto your towel and wipe your feet to remove any dirt or pebbles that may be stuck to them. Slip into your running shoes and cinch them up. Remove your helmet and grab your running hat (if applicable). If you are wearing a race belt, move your number to the front. Walk or run slowly to the exit from T2 where the run leg begins. This is generally not the same as where you came off the bike and entered T2. Be sure you know where the T2 exit is before the race begins.

The Run

Head out onto the run course, paying close attention to how you feel. Should you find yourself breathing extraordinarily hard or having a higher heart rate than you're used to while running, slow down and walk for a while. Otherwise, continue to run slowly and steadily while watching for race officials who will direct you through the course. Be aware that you may come to an intersection without an official or a police officer, so look for signs or arrows on the road. Ultimately, you need to know the course.

When you come to an aid station there will be volunteers handing out cups of water and sports drinks. Walk through each aid station and take a cup of sports drink. Don't try to run and drink; just walk so you can get most of it down. Then continue running.

It's okay to walk at any time. This is your first triathlon, so have fun. There is no need to push yourself to your limits today. Look around and enjoy the experience of running in a triathlon with others who share your passion for health and fitness.

The Finish

As the finish line comes into view, you'll undoubtedly begin to speed up. Crossing under the finish banner, slow to a walk. A race volunteer will direct you through the finish chute. At the end of the chute another race official will detach the perforated portion of your paper race number. These volunteers won't know what your time was. Your time and place overall and in your age group will be posted later. It will be easy to tell where this posting is located, as there will be lots of triathletes crowding around that area looking for their results.

AFTER THE RACE

You did it! You finished your first triathlon and you're grinning ear to ear! But you don't really feel like celebrating much right now; you are tired and want to get off your legs. It's best to walk around for a few minutes to keep the blood moving and allow for a gradual cooldown. Five minutes or so should do it. You might walk over to where the post-race goodies are available for entrants and get something to eat and drink. If you do not feel like eating much right now, look for a sports drink or eat something soft, like a banana. Getting in a few calories now will help you feel better later on.

Now you can go sit down with friends and family and tell them about your great experience. If you wore a stopwatch on your wrist during the race and pushed the lap button at the ends of the swim, bike, and run, you will be able now to recall the time splits for each leg of the race. You may be surprised to find that you went faster for each leg of the race than you had ever done in practice. It's amazing what extra rest leading up to a race and strong motivation on race day can do for performance.

Hang around afterward for the awards ceremony. It may not begin until an hour or so after you finish, but the wait for the ceremony is worth it. While you wait, try eating a bit. If your stomach is still a little queasy, don't force it down. Just continue sipping sports drinks or soft drinks. Once the ceremony begins, it goes quickly. Usually the top three in each age group are announced and called forward to receive their awards. When they come to your age group, listen for the times of the top finishers. It's remarkable how fast the top triathletes are in each age group.

If you didn't get to see your results at the race, go to the triathlon's official web site the next day to view the posting. There you can find your name and see what your time splits were for each leg of the race. You might want to print this and keep it for future reference. As you move on in the sport, this will be your reference point. You're a triathlete now!

EPILOGUE

My nearly 3-year-old granddaughter, Keara, loves going to the swimming pool and riding her tricycle, and she runs everywhere with enthusiasm. None of these things are "practice" for her—they are who she is. She doesn't compartmentalize the things she does. Eventually, I expect she will learn to divide the day into hours, minutes, and seconds instead of seeing it all as fun. That's too bad. Life is most enjoyable when it's free-form. I think that's one reason we look forward to our annual vacations—there are no, or at least fewer, constraints on how we spend our days. There is no routine.

Routines are not bad in and of themselves, however. If you followed a training plan in Chapter 9, that routine is what got you ready for your first triathlon. The typical triathlete's daily routine revolves around working out—perhaps even two or three times on some days. It takes a good measure of commitment to do this. Some of your friends may already be amazed at your dedication to finishing a triathlon. If you are now fully hooked on triathlon, as I hope you are, then *they ain't seen nothin' yet.*

YOUR NEXT TRIATHLON

You've probably started thinking about your next race goal. That could be to race at the same distance but faster. Or perhaps you're thinking about trying a longer race such as an Olympic-distance, a half-Ironman, or an Ironman triathlon. Races at the half- and full-Ironman distances take more than six hours to finish (17 hours is the cutoff for Ironman) and should not be embarked upon lightly. I suggest you keep them in the back of your mind and occasionally compare where you are in the sport with what you think it will take to reach such a goal.

To achieve any of these triathlon goals will require you not only to follow a routine, but even to be a bit obsessive about it, which will keep you on track for even greater fitness and self-fulfillment. But when we allow obsession to take the fun out of it, we diminish who we are. Swimming, biking, and running should be fun, not tasks to be completed and checked off. You should be following the triathlon lifestyle because you love it, not just because you've set a goal.

THE TAO TRIATHLETE

The Chinese have a word for what they do in life that is fulfilling—*tao*, or "the path." The tao triathlete exercises and trains to be a better athlete, not to go faster. Faster comes with following the path of complete devotion and unwavering focus. The tao archer spends hours completely focused on sending arrows at the target—not to see how many bull's-eyes he can make, but rather to better understand himself. The target is not an object related to scoring. It's a part of who he is.

Many triathletes want to "win" the workout. They do it only to beat their training partners, to improve on their "numbers," or to push themselves to their limits—and then check it off in their training logs. Their youthful love for and fascination with the sport are eventually displaced by disdain. The tao triathlete allows the workout to happen and sees the pool, the bike path, and the road merely as extensions of his or her life, to be accepted and enjoyed for what they are. Focusing externally on the clock or on others for every workout will eventually detract from the fun of exercise. Enjoyment and longevity in the sport come from making triathlon your lifestyle, not a mission to be accomplished.

CONSISTENCY AND MODERATION

Exercise is an end in itself. It is not merely a way of getting faster or going farther. These things will happen if you let them and remain consistent. There will be days, however, when you just don't feel like swimming, biking, or running. That's to be expected and is part of what makes you human. Missing a workout does not mean you are no longer a triathlete. Frequently missing lots of workouts does. Consistency is key to fulfillment in triathlon.

The other key to fulfillment is moderation. Do not seek your physical limits on a daily basis. Rather, gently progress toward your goals with small steps. Doing otherwise results in injury, overtraining, illness, or burnout. Always. If one of these crops up it's because you were trying to make fitness happen rather than *allowing* it to happen.

If your goals fit into your life you will train happily and with consistency because it's enjoyable. Enjoyment will also come from moderation. Enjoyment is why you do triathlons. You're not getting paid for this. Do it simply because it's fun.

THE NEW PATH

This book was only a tool in helping you finish your first triathlon. You are completely responsible for the achievement. You had to get yourself out of bed to do workouts while others slept. You changed the way you eat. You dedicated several hours a week to swimming, biking, and running. Your lifestyle has changed. In many ways you are now a new person—a triathlete.

You started reading this book to help you finish a triathlon. Now that you have done that, you can go back to your former lifestyle, or you can continue on the path you've started down. The choice is yours.

APPENDIX A
Workouts

SWIM WORKOUTS

The intensity of the following workouts is determined by five zones of perceived exertion, based on your breathing and effort:

Zone 1 Very easy effort with comfortably light breathing

Zone 2 Easy effort with increased breathing volume

Zone 3 Moderately hard effort with somewhat labored breathing

Zone 4 Hard effort with labored breathing

Zone 5 Very hard effort with panting

The workouts are written so that yards or meters can be used, depending on your pool's measurement. For simplicity, the distances specified are in meters (m).

SPRINT-DISTANCE WORKOUTS

Swim Workout #1   Total: 10 min.

Swim one length (25 m) of the pool, concentrating on your swim stroke mechanics. The effort should be low (zones 1–2). Stop and rest at the wall for 30–45 seconds. Swim back to the other wall and rest again. Continue this for 10 minutes.

Swim Workout #2   Total: 15 min.

Swim one length (25 m) of the pool, concentrating on your swim stroke mechanics. The effort should be low (zones 1–2). Stop and rest at the wall for 30–45 seconds. Swim back to the other wall and rest again. Continue this for 15 minutes.

Swim Workout #3   Total: 15 min.

Swim as far as you can without stopping or allowing your stroke mechanics to break down, no longer than 400 m. Keep the effort low (zones 1–2). Rest for 1 minute or so at the wall at the end of your nonstop swim.

For the remainder of the 15 minutes, continuously swim intervals of one length (25 m) with good form in zones 2–3, resting 30–45 seconds at the wall after each interval.

Swim Workout #4   Total: 15 min.

Swim 100 m in zone 1, focusing on stroke mechanics. Rest 30–45 seconds.

Swim 75 m with good form in zone 2. Rest 30–45 seconds.

Swim 50 m with good form in zone 2. Rest 30–45 seconds.

For the remainder of the 15 minutes, continue repeating this last interval (50 m) with good form in zone 2, followed by 30–45 seconds of rest at the wall after each swim.

Swim Workout #5   Total: 15 min.

Swim 100 m in zone 1, focusing on stroke mechanics. Rest 30–45 seconds.

Swim 4 sets of 25 m with good form in zone 3. Rest 30–45 seconds between intervals.

For the remainder of the 15 minutes, repeat the 25-m swim with good form in zone 1, followed by 30–45 seconds of rest at the wall after each interval.

Swim Workout #6   Total: 500 m

Swim 100 m in zone 1.

Swim 400 m nonstop in zones 2–3. Time yourself.

Swim Workout #7   Total: 30–60 min.

Swim with your masters swim team. Ask the instructor on the deck for feedback on your technique. If no masters group is available, swim your own endurance-oriented workout, always concentrating on good form. An endurance workout should have long sets (200 m or more) with short recoveries (less than 20 seconds). The intensity of these long intervals should be zones 3–4.

Swim Workout #8   Total: 1,300 m

This workout is for an experienced swimmer.

Warm-up: 50-m swim in zone 1, 50-m kick in zone 1, 100-m pull in zone 2, 100-m swim in zone 2.

Swim 4 sets of 100 m in zone 3. Rest 10 seconds between intervals.

Rest for 1 minute.

Swim 4 sets of 100 m with each one slightly faster than the previous one, but all below zone 5. Rest 10 seconds between intervals.

Rest for 1 minute.

Cool down with a 200-m swim in zone 1.

You may vary this workout by changing the 4 sets of 100-m swims to 8 sets of 50-m swims, 2 sets of 200-m swims, or some other pattern.

OLYMPIC-DISTANCE WORKOUTS

Swim Workout #9   Total: 20 min.

Swim one length (25 m) of the pool, concentrating on your swim stroke mechanics. The effort should be low (zones 1–2). Stop and rest at the wall for 30–45 seconds. Swim back to the other wall and rest again. Continue this for 20 minutes.

Swim Workout #10   Total: 30 min.

Swim one length (25 m) of the pool, concentrating on your swim stroke mechanics. The effort should be low (zones 1–2). Stop and rest at the wall for 30–45 seconds. Swim back to the other wall and rest again. Continue this for 30 minutes.

Swim Workout #11   Total: 30 min.

Start by swimming as far as you can without stopping or allowing your stroke mechanics to break down, no longer than 800 m. Keep the effort low—zones 1–2. Rest for 1 minute or so at the wall at the end of your nonstop swim.

For the remainder of the 30 minutes, continuously swim intervals of one length (25 m) with good form in zones 2–3, resting 30–45 seconds at the wall after each interval.

Swim Workout #12   Total: 40 min.

Swim 3 sets of 50 m in zone 1, focusing on stroke mechanics. Rest 30–45 seconds after each 50.

Swim 300 m with good form in zone 2. Rest 30–45 seconds.

Swim 200 m with good form in zone 2. Rest 30–45 seconds.

Swim 100 m with good form in zone 2. Rest 30–45 seconds.

For the remainder of the 40 minutes, continuously swim intervals of one length (25 m) with good form in zone 3, resting 30–45 seconds at the wall after each interval.

Swim Workout #13   Total: 45 min.

Swim 4 sets of 50 m in zone 1, focusing on stroke mechanics. Rest 30–45 seconds after each 50.

Swim 4 sets of 50 m with good form in zone 3. Rest 30–45 seconds between intervals.

Swim 400 m in zone 2. Rest for 30–45 seconds.

Swim 300 m in zone 2. Rest for 30–45 seconds.

Swim 200 m in zone 2. Rest for 30–45 seconds.

For the remainder of the 45 minutes, repeat the one-length (25-m) swim with good form in zone 1, followed by 30–45 seconds of rest at the wall after each.

Swim Workout #14   Total: 1,050 m

Warm up by swimming 4 sets of 50 m in zone 1. Make each interval slightly faster than the previous one. But do not go so fast that your good form breaks down. Rest 30–45 seconds after each interval.

Swim 2 sets of 400 m nonstop in zones 2–3. Rest for 30 seconds after each swim. Time yourself on the 400s. Try to make the second one a little faster than the first.

Cool down with an easy swim of 50 m, focusing on good technique.

BIKE WORKOUTS

The intensity of the following workouts is determined by five zones of perceived exertion, based on your breathing and effort:

Zone 1 Very easy effort with comfortably light breathing

Zone 2 Easy effort with increased breathing volume

Zone 3 Moderately hard effort with somewhat labored breathing

Zone 4 Hard effort with labored breathing

Zone 5 Very hard effort with panting

SPRINT-DISTANCE WORKOUTS

Bike Workout #1   Total: 20 min.

This ride is best done on a mostly flat course or on an indoor trainer.

Warm up for 5 minutes, gradually increasing the intensity from zone 1 to zone 2.

Stay mostly in zone 2 throughout the remainder of the ride (10 minutes). Concentrate on your pedaling cadence (count every revolution of your right foot for 1 minute). If your cadence is below 80 rpm on a flat stretch of road, shift to a lower (easier) gear. Every time you encounter a small hill or headwind, shift to a lower (easier) gear to maintain 80–90 rpm. Shift to a higher (harder) gear on downhills.

If on an indoor trainer, play with the gears, shifting frequently, and notice how your cadence changes and how you can make adjustments to get it back to 80–90 rpm. Cool down in zone 1 for 5 minutes.

Bike Workout #2   Total: 20 min.

This workout is best done on an indoor trainer, as it's a bit risky on the road.

Warm up for 5 minutes, building from zone 1 to zone 2.

Unclip your left foot from the pedal and place it on a chair or a box next to the bike. Then, with the bike in a low and easy gear, pedal with your right leg. You'll find that at the top of the pedal stroke there is a "dead" spot that is a bit difficult to pedal through. Focus on this dead spot to smooth it out. At first you will last only a few seconds with one leg as it fatigues quickly. Change legs when this happens.

After you've done each leg individually, clip in both feet and pedal normally for several minutes before repeating the single-leg drills.

Continue this pattern of right leg–left leg–both legs several times. Over time you will become more efficient at the top of the stroke and be able to pedal longer before tiring. This is a sign that your transitions are improving. Strive for 2-minute single-leg intervals.

Allow 5 minutes at the end for easy pedaling (zone 1) to cool down.

Bike Workout #3   Total: 30 min.

Ride on a mostly flat course or on an indoor trainer.

Warm up for 10 minutes.

Concentrate on the 9-to-3 drill. Think of the pedal stroke as being the face of a clock, with 12 o'clock at the top and 6 o'clock at the bottom. When the crank arms are parallel to the ground, the forward foot is in the 3 o'clock position and the back foot is at 9 o'clock. What you want to do in this drill is to feel as if you are moving your rear foot straight forward from 9 to 3 on the clock face without ever going through 12. Obviously you are, but by firing the muscles this way you train them to transition smoothly. Every minute or so, think about pedaling this way for several seconds. Take a mental break and then do it again. Repeat this frequently throughout the ride. Leave the last 5 minutes for an easy cooldown in zone 1.

Bike Workout #4   Total: 40 min.

Ride on a mostly flat course or on an indoor trainer.

Warm up for 10 minutes.

Concentrate repeatedly on the shoe-top drill. As you are pedaling, try to keep your foot against the top inside of the shoe and avoid touching the bottom inside of the shoe for several minutes. This drill emphasizes all parts of the pedal stroke except the downstroke, which is the easy part.

Leave the last 10 minutes for an easy cooldown in zone 1.

Bike Workout #5   Total: 40 min.

Ride on a mostly flat course or on an indoor trainer.

Warm up for 10 minutes.

Do the toe-touch drill several times. As your foot approaches the 12 o'clock position, try to touch your toes to the front end of your shoe. Make sure your heel is slightly higher than the ball of your foot when doing this.

Leave the last 10 minutes for an easy cooldown in zone 1.

Bike Workout #6   Total: 40 min. (sprint), 60 min. (Olympic)

Ride on a mostly flat course or on an indoor trainer.

Warm up for 10 minutes.

Concentrate on the spin-up drill. Shift to a lower (easier) gear and gradually increase your cadence for about *20–30 seconds* until you start to bounce on the saddle. At that point reduce your cadence slightly until you stop bouncing, and pedal as smoothly as you can for several seconds. Relax your hands and face as you do this. Then shift to a slightly higher (harder) gear and pedal normally for a few minutes. Repeat this drill several times. Over time your comfortable cadence range will increase.

Leave the last 10 minutes for an easy cooldown in zone 1.

Bike Workout #7   Total: 30 min.

Ride on a mostly flat course or on an indoor trainer.

Warm up for 10 minutes.

Concentrate on the pedal-mash drill. Shift to a higher (harder) gear, one that keeps your cadence between 50 and 60 rpm (you may need to count every time your right foot goes down for 1 minute). For 10 seconds, stay seated and drive the pedals down with a lot of effort at this low cadence. Then shift back to a normal gear and pedal easily at a comfortably high cadence for 1 minute and 50 seconds.

Repeat this drill 4 more times. In other words, do one mash drill every 2 minutes. *Do not do this drill if you have sensitive knees.* Instead, ride in zone 2 for 10 minutes.

Leave the last 10 minutes for an easy cooldown in zone 1.

Bike Workouts

Bike Workout #8   Total: 30 min.

Ride on a course with lots of short hills. The experienced rider may make this workout 60 minutes or longer.

Warm up for 10 minutes.

Climb several hills, staying seated and keeping your cadence above 70 rpm (you may need to count every time your right foot goes down for 1 minute). A variation on this workout is to do 3–5 repeats on a hill that takes about 2 minutes to climb. *Do not do this workout if you have sensitive knees.* Instead, ride in zone 2.

Leave the last 5–10 minutes for an easy cooldown in zone 1.

Bike Workout #9   Total: 40 min.

Ride on a mostly flat course or on an indoor trainer. Stay in zones 1 and 2 for the entire ride. Your cadence should be comfortably high.

Bike Workout #10   Total: 60 min.

Ride on a mostly flat course or on an indoor trainer. Stay in zones 1 and 2 for the entire ride. Your cadence should be comfortably high.

Bike Workout #11   Total: 50+ min.

Ride on a mostly flat course or on an indoor trainer.

Warm up for 15–20 minutes, building intensity from zone 1 to zone 2.

Then ride for 20 minutes steady in zone 3. (An experienced rider may do 3 or 4 of these 20-minute intervals.)

Cool down in zone 1 for about 10 minutes at a comfortably high cadence.

Bike Workout #12   Total: 60+ min.

Ride on a mostly flat course or on an indoor trainer.

Warm up for 10–20 minutes, building intensity from zone 1 to zone 2.

Then ride for 30 minutes steady in zone 3. (An experienced cyclist can do 3 repeats of 30-minute zone 3 intervals with each rising into zone 4 in the last 10 minutes.)

Cool down in zone 1 for 5–10 minutes at a comfortably high cadence.

Bike Workout #13   Total: 90 min.

This is a workout for an experienced cyclist. Ride in zones 1 and 2, with decidedly more time in zone 2, on a mostly flat course or on an indoor trainer.

Bike Workout #14   Total: 2 hr.

This is a workout for an experienced cyclist. Ride in zones 1 and 2 on a mostly flat course or on an indoor trainer. Get at least half the ride in zone 2.

Bike Workout #15   Total: 60 min.

This is a workout for an experienced cyclist.

Warm up for about 20 minutes.

During the warm-up, ride to a moderate-grade hill (3–5 percent grade) that takes 4–6 minutes to climb, and do 4 repeats in the aero, or triathlon, race position. Get about 20 minutes of total climbing time (including just the uphill portions in the 20 minutes). The coast-down time is your recovery. Keep your cadence above 80 rpm on the climbs.

Cool down for about 10 minutes in zone 1.

OLYMPIC-DISTANCE WORKOUTS
Bike Workout #16   Total: 40 min.

This ride is best done on a mostly flat course or on an indoor trainer.

Warm up for about 10–20 minutes, gradually increasing the intensity from zone 1 to zone 2.

Stay mostly in zone 2 throughout the remainder of the ride (15–25 minutes). Concentrate on your pedaling cadence (count every revolution of your right foot for 1 minute). If your cadence is below 80 rpm on a flat stretch of road, shift to a lower (easier) gear. Every time you encounter a small hill or headwind, shift to a lower (easier) gear to maintain 80–90 rpm. Shift to a higher (harder) gear on downhills. If on an indoor trainer, play with the gears, shifting frequently, and notice how your cadence changes when you do and how you can make adjustments to get it back to 80–90 rpm.

Cool down in zone 1 for 5 minutes.

Bike Workout #17   Total: 40 min.

This is best done on an indoor trainer, as it's a bit risky on the road.

Warm up for 5 minutes, building from zone 1 to zone 2.

Unclip your left foot from the pedal and place it on a chair or a box next to the bike. Then, with the bike in a low and easy gear, pedal with your right leg. You'll find that at the top of the pedal stroke there is a "dead" spot that is a bit difficult to pedal through. Focus on this dead spot to smooth it out. At first you will last only a few seconds with one leg as it fatigues quickly. Change legs when this happens.

After you've done each leg individually, clip in both feet and pedal normally for several minutes before repeating the single-leg drills.

Continue this pattern of right leg–left leg–both legs several times. Over time you will become more efficient at the top of the stroke and be able to pedal longer before tiring. This is a sign that your transitions are improving. Strive for 2-minute single-leg intervals.

Allow 5 minutes at the end for easy pedaling (zone 1) to cool down.

Bike Workout #18   Total: 50 min.

Ride on a mostly flat course or on an indoor trainer.

Warm up for 10 minutes.

Concentrate on the 9-to-3 drill. Think of the pedal stroke as being the face of a clock, with 12 o'clock at the top and 6 o'clock at the bottom. When the crank arms are parallel to the ground, the forward foot is in the 3 o'clock position and the back foot is at 9 o'clock. What you want to do in this drill is to feel as if you are moving your rear foot straight forward from 9 to 3 on the clock face without ever going through 12. Obviously you are, but by firing the muscles this way you train them to transition smoothly. Every minute or so, think about pedaling this way for several seconds. Take a mental break and then do it again. Repeat this frequently throughout the ride. Leave the last 5 minutes for an easy cooldown in zone 1.

Bike Workout #19   Total: 60 min.

Ride on a mostly flat course or on an indoor trainer.

Warm up for 10 minutes.

Concentrate repeatedly on the shoe-top drill. As you are pedaling, try to keep your foot against the top inside of the shoe and avoid touching the bottom inside of the shoe for several minutes. This drill emphasizes all parts of the pedal stroke except the downstroke, which is the easy part.

Leave the last 10 minutes for an easy cooldown in zone 1.

Bike Workout #20 Total: 60 min.

Ride on a mostly flat course or on an indoor trainer.

Warm up for 10 minutes.

Do the toe-touch drill several times. As your foot approaches the 12 o'clock position, try to touch your toes to the front end of your shoe. Make sure your heel is slightly higher than the ball of your foot when doing this.

Leave the last 10 minutes for an easy cooldown in zone 1.

Bike Workout #21 Total: 60 min.

Ride on a mostly flat course or on an indoor trainer.

Warm up for 10 minutes.

Concentrate on the spin-up drill. Shift to a lower (easier) gear and gradually increase your cadence for about *20–30 seconds* until you start to bounce on the saddle. At that point reduce your cadence slightly until you stop bouncing, and pedal as smoothly as you can for several seconds. Relax your hands and face as you do this. Then shift to a slightly higher (harder) gear and pedal normally for a few minutes. Repeat this drill several times. Over time your comfortable cadence range will increase.

Leave the last 10 minutes for an easy cooldown in zone 1.

Bike Workout #22 Total: 50 min.

Ride on a mostly flat course or on an indoor trainer.

Warm up for 20 minutes.

Concentrate on the pedal-mash drill. Shift to a higher (harder) gear, one that keeps your cadence between 50 and 60 rpm (you may need to count every time your right foot goes down for 1 minute). For 10 seconds, stay seated and drive the pedals down with a lot of effort at this low cadence. Then shift back to a normal gear and pedal easily at a comfortably high cadence for 1 minute and 50 seconds. Repeat this drill

8 more times. In other words, do one mash drill every 2 minutes. *Do not do this drill if you have sensitive knees.* Instead, ride in zone 2 for 18 minutes.

Leave the last 12 minutes for an easy cooldown in zone 1.

Bike Workout #23   Total: 50 min. (60 min. if experienced)

Ride on a course with lots of short hills.

Warm up for 10 minutes.

Climb several hills, staying seated and keeping your cadence above 70 rpm (you may need to count every time your right foot goes down for 1 minute). A variation on this workout is to do 3–5 repeats on a hill that takes about 2 minutes to climb. *Do not do this workout if you have sensitive knees.* Instead, ride in zone 2.

Leave the last 5–10 minutes for an easy cooldown in zone 1.

Bike Workout #24   Total: 60 min.

Ride on a mostly flat course or on an indoor trainer. Stay in zones 1 and 2 for the entire ride. Your cadence should be comfortably high.

Bike Workout #25   Total: 80 min.

Ride on a mostly flat course or on an indoor trainer. Stay in zones 1 and 2 for the entire ride. Your cadence should be comfortably high.

Bike Workout #26   Total: 70 min.

Ride on a mostly flat course or on an indoor trainer.

Warm up for 15 minutes, building intensity from zone 1 to zone 2.

Then do 2 repeats of 20-minute zone 3 intervals with 5 minutes of easy pedaling between them. An experienced rider may do 3 or 4 of these 20-minute intervals.

Cool down in zone 1 for about 10 minutes at a comfortably high cadence.

Bike Workout #27   Total: 80 min.

Ride on a mostly flat course or on an indoor trainer.

Warm up for 10 minutes, building intensity from zone 1 to zone 2.

Do 2 repeats of 30-minute zone 3 intervals with 5 minutes of recovery between them. An experienced cyclist can do 3 of these 30-minute zone 3 intervals with each rising into zone 4 in the last 10 minutes.

Cool down in zone 1 for 5 minutes at a comfortably high cadence.

Bike Workout #28   Total: 2 hr.

This is a workout for an experienced cyclist. Ride in zones 1 and 2, with decidedly more time in zone 2, on a mostly flat course or on an indoor trainer.

Bike Workout #29   Total: 2½ hr.

This is a workout for an experienced cyclist. Ride in zones 1 and 2 on a mostly flat course or on an indoor trainer. Get at least half the ride in zone 2.

Bike Workout #30   Total: 90 min.

This is a workout for an experienced cyclist.

Warm up for about 10 minutes.

Go to a moderate-grade hill (3–5 percent grade) that takes 4–6 minutes to climb, and do 6 repeats in the aero position. Get about 30 minutes of total climbing time. The coast-down time is your recovery. Keep your cadence above 80 rpm on the climbs.

Cool down for 5 minutes in zone 1.

Bike Workouts

RUN WORKOUTS

The intensity of the following workouts is determined by five zones of perceived exertion, based on your breathing and effort:

Zone 1 Very easy effort with comfortably light breathing

Zone 2 Easy effort with increased breathing volume

Zone 3 Moderately hard effort with somewhat labored breathing

Zone 4 Hard effort with labored breathing

Zone 5 Very hard effort with panting

SPRINT-DISTANCE WORKOUTS

Run Workout #1   Total: 20 min.

This walk-run session is best done on a flat, soft surface such as gravel, grass, dirt, or a track. Avoid concrete and asphalt if at all possible.

Warm up by walking briskly for 5 minutes, increasing the intensity from zone 1 to zone 2 as you progress.

Then alternate 15-second runs with 45-second walks 10 times. The walk portions are done briskly in zone 1. The runs should be zone 3 intensity.

Cool down by walking in zone 1 for 5 minutes.

Run Workout #2   Total: 20 min.

This walk-run session is best done on a flat, soft surface such as gravel, grass, dirt, or a track. Avoid concrete and asphalt if at all possible.

Warm up by walking briskly for 5 minutes, increasing the intensity from zone 1 to zone 2 as you progress.

Then alternate 30-second runs with 30-second walks for 10 times. The walk portions are done in zone 1. The runs should be zone 3 intensity.

Cool down by walking in zone 1 for 5 minutes.

Run Workout #3   Total: 20 min.

This walk-run session is best done on a flat, soft surface such as gravel, grass, dirt, or a track. Avoid hard surfaces if at all possible.

Warm up by walking briskly for 5 minutes, increasing the intensity from zone 1 to zone 2 as you progress.

Then alternate 60-second runs with 30-second walks 7 times. The walk portions are done in zone 1. The runs should be zone 3 intensity.

Cool down by walking in zone 1 for about 5 minutes.

Run Workout #4   Total: 20 min.

This walk-run session is best done on a flat, soft surface such as gravel, grass, dirt, or a track. Avoid concrete and asphalt if you can.

Warm up by alternating 1 minute of walking briskly in zone 1 with 1 minute of running in zone 2 for about 5 minutes.

Then run 10 minutes in zone 2. It's okay to stop and walk a few seconds if this seems harder than zone 2.

Cool down by walking in zone 1 for about 5 minutes.

Run Workout #5   Total: 30 min.

This walk-run session is best done on a flat, soft surface such as gravel, grass, dirt, or a track. Avoid concrete and asphalt.

Warm up by alternating 1 minute of walking briskly in zone 1 with 1 minute of running in zone 2 for about 5 minutes.

Then run 3 minutes in zone 2 and walk 1 minute in zone 1. Do this 5 times.

Cool down by walking in zone 1 for about 5 minutes.

Run Workout #6   Total: 30 min.

This walk-run session is best done on a flat, soft surface such as gravel, grass, dirt, or a track. Try not to run on concrete and asphalt.

Warm up by alternating 1 minute of walking briskly in zone 1 with 1 minute of running in zone 2 for a total of 5 minutes.

Then run 20 minutes in zone 2. It's okay to stop and walk a few seconds if this

Run Workouts

seems harder than zone 2. If your race will be on a hilly course, do this workout on hills. It's also okay to alternate walking and running on the hills.

Cool down by walking in zone 1 for about 5 minutes.

Run Workout #7   Total: 30 min.

This run is best done on a flat, soft surface such as gravel, grass, dirt, or a track. Avoid hard surfaces.

After starting very easily, run the remainder of the workout in zone 2. It's okay to stop and walk a few seconds if it seems harder than zone 2 at times. If your race will be on a hilly course, do this workout on a similar course. It's okay to alternate walking and running on the hills. How much distance did you cover in this workout? That's an indicator of how you are progressing toward the full race distance.

Run Workout #8   Total: 20 min.

This "strides" workout is best done on a flat, soft surface such as gravel, grass, dirt, or a track. Parks are excellent for this workout. Do not do this workout on concrete or asphalt.

Warm up by alternating 1 minute of walking briskly in zone 1 with 1 minute of running in zone 2 for a total of 7 minutes (the experienced runner can run for 15–20 minutes, building from zone 1 to zone 2).

Then on a flat or very slightly downhill course that is approximately 100 yards long, run 20 seconds in zone 4. Note that this is not at zone 5 (all-out effort). Hold back and concentrate on good running form, not speed. Count each time your right foot touches the ground for this 20 seconds. The number should be at least 28.

Turn around and walk back to your starting point. Do 4 of these strides. If you are taking fewer than 29 right-foot steps in 20 seconds, shorten and quicken your stride without running any harder than zone 4.

Cool down by walking or jogging in zone 1 for 5 minutes. The experienced runner can vary this workout by doing the strides uphill and may extend it to 45–60 minutes, with a longer warm-up and cooldown.

VARIATION: Do the first 2 or 3 strides barefoot (on grass only, and be sure to check for sharp objects first). When you put your shoes back on, try to run with the same good form you used when barefoot.

Run Workout #9   Total: 30–45 min.

This workout is for an experienced runner.

Build from zone 1 to zone 2 while concentrating on good running form with a high cadence (at least 28 right-foot strikes in 20 seconds).

Run Workout #10   Total: 60–75 min.

This workout is for an experienced runner.

In the first 30–45 minutes, build intensity from zone 1 to zone 2.

Run the last 30 minutes in zone 3.

Run Workout #11   Total: 45–60 min.

This workout is for an experienced runner.

Warm up for 10 minutes, building from zone 1 to zone 2.

Then on grass or on a track, run 3 minutes at your current 5K race pace, 5 times with 3-minute recovery intervals in between.

Cool down with an easy run in zone 1.

Run Workout #12   Total: 60–90 min.

This workout is for an experienced runner.

Build from zone 1 to zone 2 while concentrating on relaxed running form.

OLYMPIC-DISTANCE WORKOUTS
Run Workout #13   Total: 30 min.

This walk-run session is best done on a flat, soft surface such as gravel, grass, dirt, or a track. Avoid concrete and asphalt if at all possible.

Warm up by walking briskly for 5 minutes, increasing the intensity from zone 1 to zone 2 as you progress.

Then alternate 15-second runs with 45-second walks 20 times. The walk portions are done briskly in zone 1. The runs should be zone 3 intensity.

Cool down by walking in zone 1 for 5 minutes.

Run Workouts

Run Workout #14   Total: 30 min.

This walk-run session is best done on a flat, soft surface such as gravel, grass, dirt, or a track. Avoid concrete and asphalt if at all possible.

Warm up by walking briskly for 5 minutes, increasing the intensity from zone 1 to zone 2 as you progress.

Then alternate 30-second runs with 30-second walks 20 times. The walk portions are done in zone 1. The runs should be zone 3 intensity.

Cool down by walking in zone 1 for 5 minutes.

Run Workout #15   Total: 30 min.

This walk-run session is best done on a flat, soft surface such as gravel, grass, dirt, or a track. Avoid hard surfaces if at all possible.

Warm up by walking briskly for 5 minutes, increasing the intensity from zone 1 to zone 2 as you progress.

Then alternate 60-second runs with 30-second walks for 14 times. The walk portions are done in zone 1. The runs should be zone 3 intensity.

Cool down by walking in zone 1 for about 5 minutes.

Run Workout #16   Total: 30 min.

This walk-run session is best done on a flat, soft surface such as gravel, grass, dirt, or a track. Avoid concrete and asphalt if you can.

Warm up by alternating 1 minute of walking briskly in zone 1 with 1 minute of running in zone 2 for about 5 minutes.

Then run 20 minutes in zone 2. It's okay to stop and walk a few seconds if this seems harder than zone 2.

Cool down by walking in zone 1 for about 5 minutes.

Run Workout #17   Total: 40 min.

This walk-run session is best done on a flat, soft surface such as gravel, grass, dirt, or a track. Avoid concrete and asphalt.

Warm up by alternating 1 minute of walking briskly in zone 1 with 1 minute of running in zone 2 for about 5 minutes.

Then run 3 minutes in zone 2 and walk 1 minute in zone 1. Do this 7 times.

Cool down by walking in zone 1 for about 5 minutes.

Run Workout #18   Total: 40 min.

This walk-run session is best done on a flat, soft surface such as gravel, grass, dirt, or a track. Try not to run on concrete and asphalt.

Warm up by alternating 1 minute of walking briskly in zone 1 with 1 minute of running in zone 2 for a total of 5 minutes.

Then run 30 minutes in zone 2. It's okay to stop and walk a few seconds if this seems harder than zone 2. If your race will be on a hilly course, do this workout on hills. It's also okay to alternate walking and running on the hills.

Cool down by walking in zone 1 for about 5 minutes.

Run Workout #19   Total: 40 min.

This run is best done on a flat, soft surface such as gravel, grass, dirt, or a track. Avoid hard surfaces.

After starting very easily, run the remainder of the workout in zone 2. It's okay to stop and walk a few seconds if it seems harder than zone 2 at times. If your race will be on a hilly course, do this workout on a similar course. It's okay to alternate walking and running on the hills. How much distance did you cover in this workout? That's an indicator of how you are progressing toward the full race distance.

Run Workout #20   Total: 30 min.

This "strides" workout is best done on a flat, soft surface such as gravel, grass, dirt, or a track. Parks are excellent for this workout. Do not do this workout on concrete or asphalt.

Warm up by alternating 1 minute of walking briskly in zone 1 with 1 minute of running in zone 2 for a total of 7 minutes (the experienced runner can run for 15–20 minutes, building from zone 1 to zone 2).

Then on a flat or very slightly downhill course that is approximately 100 yards long, run 20 seconds in zone 4. Note that this is not in zone 5 (all-out effort). Hold back and concentrate on good running form, not speed. Count each time your right foot

Run Workouts

touches the ground for this 20 seconds. The number should be at least 28.

Turn around and walk back to your starting point. Do 8 of these strides. If you are taking fewer than 29 right-foot steps in 20 seconds, shorten and quicken your stride without running any harder than zone 4.

Cool down by walking or jogging in zone 1 for 5 minutes. The experienced runner can vary this workout by doing the strides uphill and may extend it to 45–60 minutes, with a longer warm-up and cooldown.

VARIATION: Do the first 2 or 3 strides barefoot (on grass only, and be sure to check for sharp objects first). When you put your shoes back on, try to run with the same good form you used when barefoot.

Run Workout #21   Total: 45–60 min.

This workout is for an experienced runner.

Build from zone 1 to zone 2 while concentrating on good running form with a high cadence (at least 28 right-foot strikes in 20 seconds).

Run Workout #22   Total: 75–90 min.

This workout is for an experienced runner.

In the first 45–60 minutes, build intensity from zone 1 to zone 2.

Run the last 30 minutes in zone 3.

Run Workout #23   Total: 45–60 min.

This workout is for an experienced runner.

Warm up for 10 minutes, building from zone 1 to zone 2.

Then on grass or on a track, run 3 minutes at your current 5K race pace, 5 times with 3-minute recovery intervals in between.

Cool down with an easy run in zone 1.

Run Workout #24   Total: 60–90 min.

This workout is for an experienced runner.

Build from zone 1 to zone 2 while concentrating on relaxed running form.

COMBINATION WORKOUTS

When combining workouts, remember that this is a good time to practice your transition area. See page 177.

SPRINT-DISTANCE WORKOUTS

Combination Workout #1   Total: bike 30 min., run 10–15 min.

Ride on a mostly flat course or on an indoor trainer.

Bike: Gradually increase the intensity from zone 1 to zone 2 as you warm up. Stay mostly in zone 2 throughout the remainder of the 30-minute ride.

Run: Quickly transition to a 10-minute (sprint) or 15-minute (Olympic) run or walk-run on a flat course in zones 1–2.

Combination Workout #2   Total: bike 40 min., run 10 min.

Ride on a mostly flat course or on an indoor trainer.

Bike: Gradually increase the intensity from zone 1 to zone 2 as you warm up. Stay mostly in zone 2 throughout the remainder of the 40-minute ride.

Run: Quickly transition to a 10-minute run or walk-run on a flat course in zones 1–2.

Combination Workout #3   Total: bike 50 min., run 10 min.

Ride on a course that is similar to the bike course in your first triathlon or on an indoor trainer.

Bike: After a 20-minute warm-up, building intensity from zone 1 to zone 2, ride for 30 minutes steady in zone 3 (an experienced cyclist can do the latter by alternating between zone 3 and zone 4 at will).

Run: Quickly transition to a 10-minute run or walk-run on a flat course in zones 1–2.

Combination Workout #4   Total: bike 50 min., run 20 min.

Ride on a course that is similar to the bike course in your first triathlon or on an indoor trainer.

Bike: Warm up for 20 minutes building intensity from zone 1 to zone 2. Ride 30 minutes steady in zone 3 (an experienced cyclist can alternate between zones 3 and 4).

Run: Quickly transition to a 20-minute run or walk-run on a flat course in zones 1–2.

OLYMPIC-DISTANCE WORKOUTS

Combination Workout #5   Total: bike 45 min., run 15 min.

Ride on a mostly flat course or on an indoor trainer.

Bike: Gradually increase the intensity from zone 1 to zone 2 as you warm up. Stay mostly in zone 2 throughout the remainder of the 45-minute ride.

Run: Quickly transition to a 15-minute run or walk-run on a flat course in zones 1–2.

Combination Workout #6   Total: bike 55 min., run 15 min.

Ride on a mostly flat course or on an indoor trainer.

Bike: Gradually increase the intensity from zone 1 to zone 2 as you warm up. Stay mostly in zone 2 throughout the remainder of the 55-minute ride.

Run: Quickly transition to a 15-minute run or walk-run on a flat course in zones 1–2.

Combination Workout #7   Total: bike 65 min., run 15 min.

Ride on a course that is similar to the bike course in your first triathlon or on an indoor trainer.

Bike: After a 20-minute warm-up, building intensity from zone 1 to zone 2, ride for 45 minutes steady in zone 3 (an experienced cyclist can do the latter by alternating between zone 3 and zone 4 at will).

Run: Quickly transition to a 15-minute run or walk-run on a flat course in zones 1–2.

Combination Workout #8   Total: bike 65 min., run 30 min.

Ride on a course that is similar to the bike course in your first triathlon or on an indoor trainer.

Bike: After a 20-minute warm-up, building intensity from zone 1 to zone 2, ride for 45 minutes steady in zone 3 (an experienced cyclist can do the latter by alternating between zone 3 and zone 4 at will).

Run: Quickly transition to a 30-minute run or walk-run on a flat course in zones 1–2.

STRENGTH WORKOUTS

Depending on your access to a gym, follow either the weighted strength workout in your training plan or the resistance exercise circuit.

WEIGHTED STRENGTH WORKOUTS
Strength Workout #1
Anatomical Adaptation (AA) Phase   Total: 45–60 min.

The purpose of the AA phase is to perfect the exercise movements while building general body strength.

Warm up by spinning on a stationary bike for 5 minutes.

Select a 30RM load (a weight you could lift only about 30 times) and do 3 sets of 20 reps each exercise (it will feel easy). Complete all 3 sets before advancing to the next exercise. Focus on doing each exercise with perfect form. Form is more important than weight loads in this phase.

	Exercise
1	leg press
2	seated row
3	chest press

Pick one based on your personal weakness—calf, knees, hamstrings:

4	heel raise
5	knee extension
6	leg curl

7	abdominal with twist
8	standing, bent-arm lat pull down

Cool down by riding a stationary bike for 5 minutes with a high cadence and a low resistance.

Strength Workouts

Strength Workout #2
Maximum Transition (MT) Phase   Total: 45–60 min.

The purpose of the first two workouts in the MT phase is to transition from lighter to heavier loads. **This is the first week of the MT phase.**

Warm up by spinning on a stationary bike for 5 minutes.

Select a 20RM load (a weight you could lift only about 20 times) and do 3 sets of 15–20 reps each. Stop each set when you feel as if you could lift the weight only one or two more times. Do *not* go to failure. Complete all 3 sets before advancing to the next exercise. Maintain good form on each rep.

	Exercise
1	leg press
2	seated row

Pick one based on your personal weakness—calf, knees, hamstrings:

4	heel raise
5	knee extension
6	leg curl

7	abdominal with twist
8	standing, bent-arm lat pull down

Note that the chest press exercise, or the push-up exercise for resistance, is not included in this phase.

Cool down by riding a stationary bike for 5 minutes with a high cadence and a low resistance.

Strength Workouts

Strength Workout #3
Maximum Transition (MT) Phase   Total: 45–60 min.

The purpose of the MT phase is to improve triathlon-specific movement strength.

This is for all weeks of the MT phase after the first week.

Warm up by spinning on a stationary bike for 5 minutes.

Select a 15RM load (a weight you could lift only about 15 times) and do 3 sets of 10–15 reps each.

Stop each set when you feel as if you could lift the weight only one or two more times. Do *not* go to failure. Complete all 3 sets before advancing to the next exercise. Maintain good form on each rep.

	Exercise
1	leg press
2	seated row

Pick one based on your personal weakness—calf, knees, hamstrings:

4	heel raise
5	knee extension
6	leg curl

7	abdominal with twist
8	standing, bent-arm lat pull down

Note that the chest press exercise, or the push-up exercise for resistance, is not included in this phase.

Cool down by riding a stationary bike for 5 minutes with a high cadence and a low resistance.

Strength Workouts

Strength Workout #4
Strength Maintenance (SM) Phase   Total: 45–60 min.

The purpose of the SM phase is to maintain the strength you have built.

Warm up by spinning on a stationary bike for 5 minutes.

Do only 2 sets with 10–15 reps of each exercise. Do the *first set* with a 20RM load (a weight you could lift 20 times). The *second set* is heavier with a 15RM load (a weight you could lift 15 times). Stop the second set when you feel as if you could lift the weight only one or two more times. Do *not* go to failure. Complete all sets before advancing to the next exercise. Maintain good form on each rep.

	Exercise
1	leg press
2	seated row

Pick one based on your personal weakness—calf, knees, hamstrings:

4	heel raise
5	knee extension
6	leg curl

7	abdominal with twist
8	standing, bent-arm lat pull down

Note that the chest press exercise, or the push-up exercise for resistance, is not included in this phase.

Cool down by riding a stationary bike for 5 minutes with a high cadence and a low resistance.

Strength Workouts

Alternate Strength Workout:
Resistance Training   Total: 30 min.

Make it your goal to perfect the exercise movements while building general body strength. Because you are not using weights, you can follow the same progression throughout your training, adding reps as you become stronger.

Warm up by spinning on a stationary bike for 5 minutes.

Complete all 3 sets before advancing to the next exercise. Stop each set when you feel as if you could do just one or two more reps. Do *not* go to failure. Focus on doing each exercise with perfect form.

	Resistance Exercise
1	one-leg squat
2	seated row with band
3	push-up

Pick one based on your personal weakness—calf, knees, hamstrings:

4	toe raises with band
5	knee extension with band
6	assisted leg curl

7	crunches with twist
8	lat pull with band

Cool down by riding a stationary bike for 5 minutes with a high cadence and a low resistance.

Strength Workouts

APPENDIX B
Gear Checklists

Following are lists of triathlon equipment that you will need or may want for your first triathlon.

MUST-HAVE GEAR

_____ Swimsuit, tri suit, or bike shorts (worn throughout the race)

_____ Run and bike shirt (may be a T-shirt)

_____ Swim goggles

_____ Swim cap (usually provided by race)

_____ Bike

_____ Bike shoes (may be running shoes)

_____ Bike helmet

_____ Bike water bottle

_____ Sports drink

_____ Running shoes

_____ Sunscreen

_____ Race instructions

_____ Race number (may be on bike and/or elastic belt, or pinned to shirt)

GOOD-TO-HAVE GEAR

_____ Wet suit (if open-water swim and allowed by the race director)

_____ Aerobars on bike

_____ Handlebar computer

_____ Lace locks or elastic laces on shoes

_____ Race belt for attaching number (number may be pinned to shirt instead)

_____ Bike pump

_____ Wrist stopwatch/heart rate monitor (with chest strap)/GPS

_____ Transition towel

_____ After-race clothing

_____ Sunglasses

_____ Cold weather gear (gloves, jacket, arm warmers, etc.)

_____ Repair kit with basic tools

HELPFUL-TO-HAVE GEAR

_____ Running shorts to wear over swimsuit on bike and run

_____ Nose clip and earplugs for swimming

_____ Running hat

_____ Nonstick cooking spray to help slip wet suit off (open-water swim)

_____ Big plastic bag to carry wet swim stuff home

_____ Spare pair of swim goggles

_____ Windbreaker for biking in case it's cold

_____ Toilet paper

_____ Plastic bag to cover saddle (in case of rain while it's racked)

_____ Transition stall marker (for example, balloon or ribbon)

_____ Socks (rolled down for easy entry in T1)

GEAR FOR DESTINATION RACES

_____ Nonperishable breakfast foods

_____ Personal pillow (if driving to race)

APPENDIX C
Triathlon Resources

TRIATHLON BOOKS

The following are popular and helpful books on triathlon. All are in print as of this writing.

Bernhardt, G. *Training Plans for Multisport Athletes*. Boulder, CO: VeloPress, 2006.

Carmichael, C. *The CTS Collection: Training Tips for Cyclists and Triathletes*. Boulder, CO: VeloPress, 2001.

Edwards, S. *The Complete Book of Triathlons*. Roseville, CA: Prima, 2001.

Edwards, S. *Triathlons for Women*, 4th ed. Boulder, CO: VeloPress, 2010.

Evans, M. *Triathlete's Edge*. Champaign, IL: Human Kinetics, 2003.

Fitzgerald, M. *Complete Triathlon Book*. New York: Warner Books, 2003.

Friel, J. *The Triathlete's Training Bible*, 3rd ed. Boulder, CO: VeloPress, 2009.

Friel, J. *Your Best Triathlon*. Boulder, CO: VeloPress, 2010.

Friel, J., and G. Byrn. *Going Long: Training for Triathlon's Ultimate Challenge*, 2nd ed. Boulder, CO: VeloPress, 2009.

Hagerman, P. *Strength Training for Triathletes*. Boulder, CO: VeloPress, 2008.

Harr, E. *Triathlon Training in Four Hours a Week*. Emmaus, PA: Rodale, 2003.

Hobson, W., C. Campbell, and M. Vickers. *Swim, Bike, Run*. Champaign, IL: Human Kinetics, 2001.

Holland, T. *The 12-Week Triathlete*, 2nd ed. Beverly, MN: Fair Winds Press, 2005.

Laughlin, T. *Triathlon Swimming Made Easy.* Goshen, NY: Total Immersion, 2002.

Mora, J. *Triathlon 101,* 2nd ed. Champaign, IL: Human Kinetics, 2009.

Murphy, T. J. *Triathlete Magazine's Guide to Finishing Your First Triathlon.* New York: Skyhorse, 2008.

Niles, R. *Time-Saving Training for Multisport Athletes.* Champaign, IL: Human Kinetics, 1997.

Pitney, D., and D. Dourney. *Triathlon Training for Dummies.* Hoboken, NJ: Wiley, 2009.

TRIATHLON WEB SITES

www.beginnertriathlete.com. A robust online community featuring training advice, athlete forums, race listings, and much more.

www.triathlete.com. This web site draws from the sport's long-standing magazine, featuring extensive coverage of professional racing plus age-group coverage and plenty of training information.

www.usatriathlon.org. This is the official web site of USA Triathlon, the governing body of the sport in the United States. It has a race calendar, information on clubs and coaches, a membership application, and updates on the sport.

www.trainingbible.com. Here you will find coaches for hire in the United States and in other countries, along with a free newsletter, free training resources, and a listing of camps and clinics.

www.trainingpeaks.com. At this interactive web site you can log your workouts online, plan your training, and analyze your performance. There is also a forum here moderated by coaches.

www.lavamagazine.com. This site's name celebrates the Ironman World Championships in Kona, Hawaii. You'll find race coverage, training information, and features on the pros, but as the name suggests, this magazine and web site are best suited for the dedicated triathlete.

www.slowtwitch.com. Slowtwitch covers a broad range of topics, including race results, product reviews, training advice, and editorial comment on the goings-on in the world of triathlon.

www.trifind.com. This is a search engine you can use to find U.S. races and to link to the races' web sites where you can register.

GLOSSARY

The following terms are used in books and magazines about triathlon and by triathletes in conversation.

Active recovery. A very easy workout intended to promote recovery from hard training. See also Passive recovery

Age group. A competitive division among the amateurs in a race, such as "female 30–34."

Age grouper. An amateur triathlete.

Aerobars. A type of bike handlebar that makes the rider more aerodynamic.

Body marking. The writing of your race number and age group on your arm and leg by a race volunteer before a triathlon.

Bonk. Extreme exhaustion, usually caused by using up most of the carbohydrates stored in your muscles.

BOP. A triathlete who usually finishes in the "back of the pack," or among the last of the entrants.

Brick. A continuous, combination workout including either the swim and bike or bike and run.

Cadence. Revolutions or cycles per minute of the swim stroke, pedal stroke, or run stride.

Cooldown. Low-intensity exercise at the end of a workout.

DNF. Abbreviation for "did not finish" in the race results.

Drafting. Swimming, biking, or running closely behind someone else to reduce effort.

Drops. The lower portion of turned-down handlebars.

Free weights. Weights that are not part of an exercise machine, such as barbells and dumbbells.

Frequency. The number of times per week that someone works out.

Half-Ironman. A triathlon with 1.2-mile swim, 56-mile bike, and 13.1-mile run portions.

Hammer. A fast, sustained effort.

Hamstring. The muscle on the back of your thigh that flexes the knee and extends the hip.

Hoods. On drop handlebars, the covers of the brake handles.

Intervals. A type of high-intensity exercise marked by short but regularly repeated periods of hard efforts separated by periods of recovery.

Ironman. A trademarked brand owned by the World Triathlon Corporation, referring to a triathlon with 2.4-mile swim, 112-mile bike, and 26.2-mile run portions.

Mash. To push a high gear on your bike.

MOP. A triathlete who usually finishes in the "middle of the pack" of entrants.

Newbie. Someone new to triathlon.

Olympic-distance race. A triathlon with 1,500-meter swim, 25-mile bike, and 6.2-mile run portions.

Passive recovery. A period of time with no workouts, intended to promote recovery from hard training; a day off from exercise. (*See also* Active recovery.)

Periodization. A method of sequentially organizing training to achieve a high level of fitness by the time of an important race.

PR. Abbreviation for "personal record"—someone's best time ever for a given swim, bike, or run distance; also sometimes referred to as "PB" for "personal best."

Quadriceps ("quads"). The large muscle in front of the thigh that straightens the knee and flexes the hip.

Repetition. The number of times a task, such as lifting a weight, is repeated.

RPM. Revolutions per minute. Same as cadence.

Set. A group of repetitions.

Singlet. A sleeveless shirt, often worn when running or biking.

Spinning. Pedaling at a high cadence or RPM.

Split. Someone's time for a given portion of the race, such as the bike split.

Sprint-distance race. A short triathlon with distances that are generally about 400–500 meters for the swim, 10–15 miles for the bike, and 3 miles for the run.

T1. Transition #1—the swim-to-bike transition.

T2. Transition #2—the bike-to-run transition.

Taper. A short period of time, generally a few days or one to two weeks, before an important race during which the amount of training done is reduced to increase rest, which produces greater fitness.

Transition. An area designated for changing from one sport to the next, such as from swim to bike (*see* T1) and bike to run (*see* T2).

Tops. The portion of the drop-down handlebars closest to the stem.

Warm-up. The period of gradually increasing intensity of exercise at the start of a workout.

Wave. A group of triathletes within a race who are started at the same time in order to prevent overcrowding on the course.

INDEX

ABOUT THE AUTHOR

Since 1980 **Joe Friel** has been training endurance athletes from all corners of the globe, including novice, elite amateur, and professional road cyclists; mountain bikers; triathletes and duathletes; national champions; world championship competitors; and an Olympian.

Joe holds a master's degree in exercise science. He is a founder and past chairman of the USA Triathlon National Coaching Commission. He has also been featured as a columnist for several magazines around the world.

Joe conducts seminars and camps throughout the world on training and racing for cyclists, multisport athletes, and coaches. He provides consulting services for corporations in the fitness industry and for the national Olympic federations. He is a cofounder of Training Peaks (trainingpeaks.com) and TrainingBible Coaching (trainingbible.com). Go to joefrielsblog.com to keep up with what's going on in the world of endurance-sport training.

As an age-group competitor, Joe is a Colorado State Masters triathlon champion and a Rocky Mountain region and Southwest region duathlon age-group champion. He also has represented the United States at the world championships several times. Currently, he enjoys competing in bike races and time trials.

Joe lives and trains in the McDowell Mountains in Scottsdale, Arizona, on the edge of the Sonoran Desert, and in the Rocky Mountains of Boulder, Colorado, the mecca of endurance-sport training. He may be reached at jfriel@trainingbible.com.